ENJOY GREAT HEALTH WHEN YOU ENTER
THE ZONE

"The hottest diet in Hollywood."
Woman's World

"If you do what Dr. Sears recommends,
you'll not only improve your health
and well-being . . . you'll also notice
how much easier it is to
connect the dots."
Bill Cosby

"Clearly distilled science and
a detailed eating plan for
peak performance."
New York Times

"*The Zone* works for me."
Cindy Crawford

WHAT TO EAT IN THE ZONE

Books by Dr. Barry Sears

The Anti-Inflammation Zone
What to Eat in the Zone
A Week in the Zone
The Omega Rx Zone
Zone Meals in Seconds
The Top 100 Zone Foods
The Soy Zone
The Anti-Aging Zone
Zone Food Blocks
Zone-Perfect Meals in Minutes
Mastering the Zone
The Zone

DR. BARRY SEARS

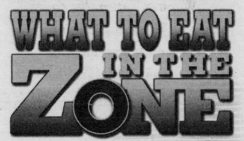

WHAT TO EAT IN THE ZONE

THE QUICK & EASY, MIX & MATCH COUNTER FOR STAYING IN THE ZONE

(Originally published as *Zone Food Blocks*)

HARPER

An Imprint of HarperCollins*Publishers*

A hardcover edition of this book was published in 1998 under the title *Zone Food Blocks* by HarperCollins/ReganBooks.

HARPERTORCH
An Imprint of HarperCollins*Publishers*
10 East 53rd Street
New York, New York 10022-5299

Copyright ©1998, 2004 by Dr. Barry Sears
ISBN: 0-06-058742-3

First HarperTorch/ReganBooks paperback printing: January 2004

HarperCollins ®, HarperTorch™, and ❤™ are trademarks of Harper-Collins Publishers Inc.

Printed in the United States of America

Visit HarperTorch on the World Wide Web at www.harpercollins.com

20 19 18 17 16 15

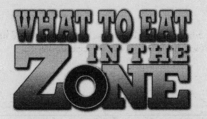

CONTENTS

ACKNOWLEDGMENTS

There are a number of people who have made this comprehensive book possible. First and foremost are my wife, Lynn Sears, and my brother, Doug Sears, who have both spent years with me in developing the concept of the Zone and the use of Zone Food Blocks. A special thanks goes to Cassie Jones for her critical comments and expert editing of this manuscript.

But the person most responsible for this book is my publisher, Judith Regan, without whose faith and belief in the Zone, this and all of the preceding Zone books may never have been written.

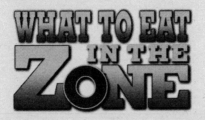

PART 1
Getting Started

PART I
Getting Started

WHAT IS THE ZONE?

What is the Zone? You have probably heard many things about it. Let me first say what the Zone is not. It is not a high-protein diet, and it is not a high-fat diet, and it is not a high-carbohydrate diet. It is, however, about moderation and balance. Specifically, it's about hormonal balance—keeping hormonal responses (and in particular, the hormone insulin) generated by the food you eat within a zone: not too high, not too low. If insulin levels are too high, you will accumulate excess stored body fat. If insulin levels are too low, your cells will starve to death. In essence, when you follow the Zone Diet you are treating food as if it were a drug, giving food the same respect that you would give any prescription drug. This is a revolutionary concept, and this is why the Zone is controversial. When viewed through this hormonal prism, food can be your greatest ally or your worst enemy; you just have to know how to play by the rules that haven't changed in 40 million years and are unlikely to change tomorrow.

WHY IS THE ZONE IMPORTANT TO YOU?

You need to be in the Zone, because your life depends on it. The Zone is about hormonal thinking and how the food you eat controls very powerful hormones that are often hundreds of times more powerful than prescription drugs. Hormones are the chemical messengers of your body. They direct every one of your body's vital systems as they can either drive your body toward illness and disease or redirect your body toward health. When they are functioning at their best, they can help your body achieve a state of wellness and optimal performance. This is what the Zone Diet is all about. Once you begin to think about food hormonally, you soon realize just how powerful a drug food actually is. This doesn't mean that food has to taste like a drug, but it does mean that it's important to realize that food can have adverse hormonal side effects, such as the overproduction of insulin.

Hormonal thinking is very different than caloric thinking. Caloric thinking can be summarized by this philosophy: "if no fat touches my lips, then no fat reaches my hips." This type of thinking has been the nutritional mantra in America for the past 15 years. During this time, fat has been made to be the villain of our society. Yet in that same 15-year period we have actually been eating less fat than ever before and, in the process, have become the fattest people on the face of the earth (1). What went wrong? Maybe fat is not the demon we have been told. This is why more and more scientists are voicing their doubts in prestigious journals like the *New England Journal of Medicine* in 1997:

"Replacement of fat by carbohydrate has not been shown to reduce the risk of coronary disease. . . ." (2)

"Beneficial effects of high-carbohydrate diets on the risk of cancer or body weight have also not been substantiated. . . ." (2)

Or other medical researchers who have stated:

"The more insulin-resistant the individual, the greater the likelihood that low-fat, high-carbohydrate diets will increase the risk factors for ischemic heart disease." (3)

How could this be if we have been told that eating a low-fat, high-carbohydrate diet is the key to better health? In essence, these respected scientists are saying the emperor (i.e., the low-fat diet, high-carbohydrate diet) has no clothes. Americans have been sold a pig in a poke for the last 15 years with the expectation that low-fat, high-carbohydrate diets would be the panacea for our health and wellness. The hormonal thinking behind the Zone explains why this hasn't happened. In fact, the general state of health in America is worse now than it was 15 years ago. Fortunately, there is a solution to this health crisis because it can be reversed with the Zone Diet.

ZONE BENEFITS

If dietary fat alone doesn't make you fat (besides not causing heart disease and cancer), then what does? One answer is excess levels of the hormone insulin. The power of the Zone is that this hormone can be controlled by the diet. The Zone is about keeping insulin in a range or zone—not too high, not too low. Not only can keeping insulin in a tight zone prevent you from gaining weight and help you to lose it, but also maintaining insulin in this same zone produces the following benefits:

- Thinking better
- Performing better
- Looking better
- Living better (and longer)

Who doesn't want to experience these benefits? Let's take them one by one.

Thinking Better

Maintaining peak mental acuity is simply a consequence of maintaining stable blood sugar levels. Blood sugar is the metabolic fuel your brain uses to maintain your mental activity. If blood sugar levels drop, then brain function (and your thinking ability) becomes compromised since your brain is running on empty. This is known as low blood sugar or hypoglycemia. As an example, think about how you feel three hours after eating a big pasta meal. You can barely keep your eyes open, and you find yourself in a dense mental fog. That's an example of low blood sugar. Should your blood sugar levels drop even lower, the brain will actually shut down and go into a coma. This commonly occurs with diabetics who inject too much insulin. Before that drastic step happens, most people will reach for some high-carbohydrate snack that will temporarily increase blood sugar levels, but this simply starts this vicious cycle over again.

What controls your blood sugar levels? It is the amount of insulin in the bloodstream. Insulin is a storage hormone. It tells your body to drive incoming macronutrients (protein, carbohydrate, and fat) into their respective sites for storage so that they can be used at some time in the future. Too much insulin, and you drive down the levels of blood sugar by sending it to the liver and muscles for storage. This is great for those organs, but not too good for the brain. When blood sugar levels drop, clear and concise thought becomes more difficult. I don't care how many Ph.D.'s you have, once low blood sugar sets in, your mental capacity drops like a stone. On the other hand, if you can maintain insulin in the Zone, then you stabilize blood sugar levels, giving you peak mental acuity for four to six hours after your last Zone meal. That's the good news. The bad news is that in order to maintain your insulin levels in that Zone, you must eat another Zone meal every four to six hours. In essence you are treating food as if it were a drug, to be taken at the right dosage and the right time.

Performing Better

The average American male or female carries more than 100,000 stored calories as fat on their body. This is a remarkable amount of energy. In fact it is equivalent to eating 1,700 pancakes for breakfast. The problem is how to access this stored energy for your daily activities. The answer is to lower elevated insulin levels to get into the Zone. Once your insulin levels are in the Zone, it's as if you have a "hormonal ATM" card that allows you to tap into those 1,700 "fat pancakes" throughout the day. On the other hand, if you have high levels of insulin, there is no way you can ever access those "fat pancakes" for energy because elevated insulin blocks the enzyme that is required for their release. And here is another bit of bad news about excess insulin. If you are exercising or doing any physical activity, realize that high levels of insulin decrease oxygen transfer to your muscle cells, thereby building up lactic acid which causes muscle fatigue. So if you want to perform better throughout the day, keep your insulin levels in the Zone.

Looking Better

The loss of excess body fat should be considered a pleasant side effect of being in the Zone. The only way you can lose this extra fat is to lower insulin. Remember insulin is a storage hormone that tells your body to hang onto all the calories it has stored. And these include fat calories stored in your adipose tissue. So in fact, it's not a matter of losing weight but losing excess body fat while retaining your lean body mass. Keep in mind it's your percent body fat that indicates how good you are going to look in a swimsuit. The reason Olympic swimmers look so good in swimsuits is that they have a low percent body fat coupled with good muscle mass. They actually weigh a lot more than a marathon runner but have a lower percent body fat. So if you want to look better, then you have to keep insulin in the Zone.

Living Better (and Longer)

Excess insulin is like a loose hormonal cannon on the deck of a ship because elevated insulin is the primary risk factor associated with heart disease, which remains the number one killer of both males and females in America. Excess insulin also decreases the efficiency of your immune system by increasing the levels of certain hormones (i.e., eicosanoids) that depress the immune system and cause silent inflammation. The underlying reason behind our declining state of health in America is the epidemic rise of silent inflammation. This is the inflammation that can't be perceived as outright pain, but it is relentless in wearing down your brain, your heart, and your immune system. Now that it can be measured for the first time, we know that it is the foundation for the development of heart disease, cancer and Alzheimer's. And the best way to accelerate silent inflammation is to eat too many carbohydrates because that increases the secretion of insulin. Excess insulin not only makes you fat and keeps you fat, but excess insulin also increases silent inflammation in your body. There lies the smoking gun between obesity and chronic disease; the increase in silent inflammation. Besides being the fattest people in the world, Americans are also the most inflamed. So, if you want to live better and longer, then it's simply a matter of keeping insulin in the Zone. On the other hand, if you don't have any desire to live better or live longer, then you can stop reading this book now.

MAKING ZONE MEALS USING
THE HAND-EYE METHOD

The preparation of Zone meals is a lot easier than you might think. All you need are your hand and your eye. That's why I call it the "hand-eye" method. At every meal, simply take your plate and divide it into three equal sections as shown in Figure 1.

**Divide your plate
into 3 sections**

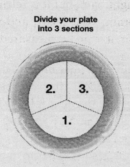

Figure 1. Empty plate divided into three equal sections

On one-third of the plate you put some low-fat protein (like chicken, fish, etc.) that is no bigger nor thicker than the palm of your hand. This will be about 3 oz. for a typical female and 4 oz. for the typical male as shown in Figure 2.

On the other two-thirds of the plate, you fill (i.e., supersize) it until it's overflowing with carbohydrates, such as non-starchy vegetables and fruit, as shown in Figure 3.

Finally, you add a dash (that's a small amount) of heart-healthy monounsaturated fat like olive oil,

Fill ⅓ with low-fat protein

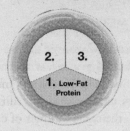

(A typical portion fits in your palm and is no thicker)

Figure 2. One-third of plate with low-fat protein

slivered almonds or even guacamole. That's it. You just constructed a Zone meal that will stabilize insulin (and blood sugar) for the next four to six hours. The only trick is to do it the best you can at every meal since you don't get brownie points from one meal to the next. But that also means no matter how bad

Supersize the remainder of your plate with vegetables and fruits

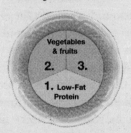

Finally, add a dash of heart-healthy fat (Olive Oil, Avocado, or Slivered Almonds)

Figure 3. Completely filled plate

your last meal, your next meal can bring you back to the Zone.

Frankly if that was all you needed, this would be a very short book. Actually there is a little more to it. To master the Zone, you have to learn what (1) carbohydrates really are, and (2) how the volumes of different food ingredients can be radically different even though they contain the same number of calories.

Let's answer the first question; what is a carbohydrate? Most people know that pasta and sweets are carbohydrates. On the other hand, most Americans are positively amazed to find out that fruits and vegetables are also carbohydrates. They usually think of them as something from the planet Uranus. I believe this is one of the reasons that Americans are so confused about what to eat because we don't have any idea what we are eating.

Now let's tackle the second question about the volumes of different food ingredients. For protein and fat this is pretty simple. Most protein choices have about the same density of protein so all you have to do is to use your palm to measure the amount you need at any meal. The same is true of fats; except they are usually so concentrated you only need a small amount of added fat at any one meal (that's why you use only a dash). It's the carbohydrates that cause all the confusion. Some carbohydrates, such as grains and starches, are very dense sources of carbohydrates, whereas some carbohydrates, such as vegetables, are very low in carbohydrates. This is why some nine years ago I invented the concept of Zone

Food Blocks to help put carbohydrates (and also protein and fat) on a common playing ground to make it easier to hormonally balance your plate at every meal.

WHAT ARE ZONE FOOD BLOCKS?

Before getting to Zone Food Blocks, you need to learn a bit about nutrition first. For starters, just remember this little rhyme which says: Protein moves around, and carbohydrates grow in the ground.

Fish move around so they must be protein. Chickens move around, so they must be protein also. So far so good. Now here's the hard part: what's a carbohydrate? Most people will immediately say pasta. Pasta comes from wheat which grows in the ground, so it must be a carbohydrate. But then broccoli also grows in the ground and so do apple trees. The fact that vegetables and fruits are also carbohydrates remains a startling revelation to most Americans.

And fat? We have been told that it is the evil incarnate. But actually, there are good fats and bad fats. Bad fats include saturated fat and artificial trans fatty acids. Everyone agrees these should be a minor part of your diet. On the other hand, good fats include monounsaturated fats (like olive oil) and Omega-3 fats (like fish oil). As I will explain later, adding the right type of fat to each meal and snack is critically important for the success of the Zone Diet.

Once you have a clearer conception of what protein,

carbohydrate, and fats actually are (and there will always be some exceptions) then you have to deal with the fact that different food items contain at least one (if not more) of these macronutrients (i.e., protein, carbohydrate, and fat) in different densities even if the foods are related to one another. As an example, pasta and broccoli are both carbohydrates. But one cup of cooked pasta contains the same number of carbohydrates as 12 cups of steamed broccoli. Although there will be an obvious difference in the total volume of these items on your plate, they both contain the same amount of carbohydrates. Likewise, 4 ounces of chicken breast will contain the same amount of protein as 12 ounces of tofu. And that's why I developed Zone Food Blocks—so that you can compare the amount of a particular macronutrient in any food ingredient with the quantity of the same macronutrient in another food ingredient. Essentially, using the Zone Food Blocks, all the calculations are done for you. You no longer think about grams or calories but simply the amount of Zone Food Blocks contained in a typical food ingredient. Since most people are not likely to eat more than 20 food items in their entire lives, remembering the sizes of your favorite foods in terms of Zone Food Blocks becomes easier than remembering family birthdays. And because the Zone Food Block system normalizes nutrient density between many foods, you'll have an easy time making Zone meals.

Now let me show how each of these Zone Food Blocks is actually calculated and then why they let you make Zone meals with ease.

CARBOHYDRATES

Zone carbohydrate blocks are complicated by two factors. The first is the fiber content of the food, and the second is the food's water content. Carbohydrate Zone blocks are based upon the amount of carbohydrate that actually enters the bloodstream and thus stimulates the release of insulin. Since fiber doesn't enter the bloodstream, you have to subtract out the fiber content of any food in order to determine the amount of insulin-stimulating carbohydrate actually in that food. This is why I define one carbohydrate block as 9 grams of insulin-stimulating carbohydrate. Now you can understand why 3 cups of steamed broccoli has the same amount of insulin-stimulating carbohydrate as ¼ cup of cooked pasta. Although each contains the same amount of insulin-stimulating carbohydrate, the broccoli has lots of water and lots of fiber, whereas the pasta doesn't. The water content also explains why it takes nearly two heads of lettuce to make one carbohydrate block. The lettuce is virtually all water with some fiber to hold it together. That's why it takes a lot of vegetables to make up one carbohydrate Zone Food Block. Fruits generally have less water and less fiber than vegetables, so they are intermediate in volume when calculated in terms of Zone Food Blocks. Finally, grains and starches have very little fiber and virtually no water, so they are extremely carbohydrate-dense, and, as a result, it takes very small amounts of them to constitute one carbohydrate Zone Food Block.

While virtually no protein contains carbohydrates (except for some dairy products and tofu), some carbohydrates do contain small amounts of protein. Moreover, the amounts of protein are very low in comparison to the amount of carbohydrate also contained within the same carbohydrate. Another complicating factor is that the high-fiber content of vegetables prevents a good chunk of that protein from being absorbed. Therefore, you have to reduce the actual amount of protein contained in a carbohydrate source (like beans) to reflect the amount of protein that will be absorbed. On average only 70 to 75 percent of the vegetable protein will be absorbed. I have taken this correction factor into account when calculating the number of protein Zone blocks found in vegetable sources. Although I have incorporated these correction factors, frankly it is just easier to treat vegetables as a great carbohydrate source and plan to get your protein elsewhere. (Note for vegetarians: There are excellent sources of protein-rich vegetarian sources listed in the Top Zone Food Ingredients, Part II.)

Being aware of the number of carbohydrate blocks in a meal is critical on the Zone Diet because carbohydrates are very potent stimulators of insulin. The Zone Diet is all about insulin control, so any excess consumption of carbohydrates in a meal is the real enemy of the Zone concept. Unfortunately, as if working with carbohydrates wasn't already tricky enough, you also have to take into account the concepts known as the glycemic index and the glycemic load.

The glycemic index of a carbohydrate measures the rate at which a carbohydrate enters the bloodstream. The faster the carbohydrate enters the bloodstream, the more insulin is secreted. Some simple carbohydrates, such as fructose, enter the bloodstream very slowly, while some complex carbohydrates, such as bread or potatoes, enter the bloodstream very quickly. The Zone Diet is based upon hormonal thinking which strives to keep insulin within a discrete zone throughout the day. Therefore, a Zone meal is not based on whether a carbohydrate is simple or complex but how that carbohydrate will affect insulin production. This is why I like to use the term glycemic load to describe Zone meals. The glycemic load of any carbohydrate is defined as the amount of carbohydrate in a typical serving size times the glycemic index of that carbohydrate.

Glycemic Load = Glycemic Index of a Carbohydrate × Grams of that Carbohydrate in a Serving Size

Understanding the concept of the glycemic load means that having small amounts of high-glycemic load carbohydrates (like bread, pasta or starches) at a meal is okay as long as most of the carbohydrates in that same meal are coming from low-glycemic load carbohydrates, such as fruits and vegetables. This ensures that the overall composite glycemic load of a meal is not high enough to overstimulate insulin release. Let me give you an example. Black beans

---

have a low glycemic index, so that should be good for the Zone Diet. Unfortunately, they have a very high amount of total carbohydrates in a small volume. This means you can't eat massive amounts of black beans without causing a significant increase in the glycemic load of a meal. In other words, go easy on eating too many carbohydrates.

The reason the concept of the glycemic load is so important to the Zone Diet is that it predicts the impact of the carbohydrate ingredients on insulin secretion. This is why Harvard Medical School has shown that the higher the daily glycemic load, the greater the likelihood of developing obesity, type 2 diabetes, and heart disease (4) along with increasing the levels of inflammation in your body (5). As you will see in Part II, the top carbohydrate choices for making Zone meals are all low glycemic load carbohydrates.

FAT

Ironically, although the role of fat has been scorned for the past 15 years, it is one of the most important components of the Zone Diet. Why? There are several hormonal reasons that no one ever anticipated as we began our national fat phobia in the 1980s. First, fat supplies essential fatty acids to your diet. These fats are known as polyunsaturated fats and can be categorized in two distinct classes: omega-6 and omega-3 fats. Without these essential fatty acids, your body can't make another group of exceptionally powerful hormones called eicosanoids. These hormones exert a significant control on your brain, heart and immune system by controlling the levels of inflammation. Second, fat slows down the rate of entry of any carbohydrate into the bloodstream which further reduces insulin secretion. Third, fat causes the release of a hormonal signal from the gut to tell the brain to stop eating.

Finally, fat makes food taste better. Before you get too excited, let me tell you that like carbohydrates, not all fat is the same. In fact, there are some fats that you definitely want to minimize on the Zone Diet. The first of these is saturated fat. These are the fats that are solid at room temperature. Not surprisingly, excess consumption of saturated fat tends to make your cell membranes have a fluidity similar to molasses. As a result, the receptors for insulin don't work as well, and this forces your body to make even more insulin in order to drive nutrients into cells. And as you now know, the more insulin you make, the fatter you become. Another group of fats to be avoided are called trans fatty acids. These are artificial fats that have been developed by the food industry to improve the shelf life of processed foods. If you see the designation "partially hydrogenated vegetable oil" on a food label, you know it contains these trans fatty acids. The final group of fats you want to moderate are called omega-6 essential fatty acids. Although these are critical for human health (because they are the building blocks for certain types of eicosanoids), an excess of omega-6 essential fatty acids can increase the levels of inflamation in your body. By eating low-fat protein, you will consume more than adequate amounts of omega-6 essential fats.

So when you add fat to your diet (and on the Zone Diet you will), you want it to come from either mono-unsaturated fats (like olive oil, slivered almonds, and avocados) or omega-3 fatty acids, such as those found in cold-water fish. It should be noted that fish is the only source of protein that is rich in omega-3 fatty acids, while simultaneously low in omega-6 fatty acids. This is one reason why a high intake of fish in your diet or taking fish supplements is so protective against heart disease (6, 7).

And before you start thinking that the Zone Diet is a high-fat diet, let me point out that a Zone Fat Food Block contains only 3 grams of fat, which isn't very much. While fat is important to the Zone Diet, it is not a diet built upon fat gluttony.

PROTEIN

One Zone block of protein equals 7 grams of protein. Don't confuse this with the actual weight of the protein. Most animal protein is found in muscle tissue, and much of that muscle weight is water. As an example, 1 oz. of chicken breast is approximately 28 grams of total weight, but it contains only 7 grams of protein with the rest being primarily water and small amounts of fat. Using the Zone Food Block method, 1 oz. of chicken breast would equal 1 protein block.

1 oz. of chicken breast = 7 g of protein
7 g protein/7g of protein per block = 1 protein block

Some sources of protein, however, contain lots of fat and very little protein. A good example is bacon. To get the same amount of protein as found in 1 oz. of low-fat chicken breast, you would have to consume 3 ounces of bacon. Unfortunately, that amount of bacon would also contain five times as much fat. Obviously, bacon is not a very good source of protein but a tremendous source of fat (and bad fat at that). Not only is bacon a high-fat source of protein but also most of the fat is saturated. Two strikes against bacon. So you can see that bacon is obviously not a high priority item on the Zone Diet.

So here is your summary of Zone Food Blocks: Carbohydrates rarely contain any significant amounts of fat, so consider them to be fat-free. They also contain very small amounts of protein relative to the amount of carbohydrate. So, just to make it simple, consider them also to be protein-free. On the other hand, protein almost always contains some fat. A good rule to follow is that every Zone block of low-fat protein will contain about one-half block of a "hidden" fat. As an example, take chicken breast in which 1 oz. of meat will contain one block of protein (7 grams) and less than one-half block of fat (1.4 grams). Because I have rounded all the Zone blocks to the nearest whole number, consider low-fat protein sources to have essentially zero fat blocks.

USING ZONE FOOD BLOCKS

All you have to do is to keep the balance of protein, carbohydrate, and fat blocks in 1:1:1 balance at every meal and snack. You have an infinite number of choices, all based on the foods you like to eat and, therefore, will eat.

Using the Zone Food Block method makes constructing Zone meals easy. You simply keep the number of protein blocks equal to the number of carbohydrate blocks at every meal and snack. As I explained above, although fat has no effect on the hormone insulin, it does have the benefit of (1) making food taste better, (2) slowing down the rate of entry of any carbohydrate into the bloodstream and therefore lowering the insulin response, and (3) sending a hormonal off signal to the brain that says "stop eating." These are three good reasons why you add extra fat blocks to every meal, especially if they are good fats. Every Zone meal should consist of equal numbers of protein, carbohydrate, and fat blocks. It's that simple.

The typical female will need about three Zone blocks of each carbohydrate, protein, and fat at each meal, whereas the typical male will need four Zone blocks of each at every meal. I have found that it may take about two weeks to get the hang of this program as you train your eyes to recognize what a Zone Food Block of your favorite food items actually looks like. I suggest that you go out and buy an inexpensive scale to weigh your protein and a set of inexpensive measuring cups to determine what volumes your carbohydrates actually take up. Once you learn to eyeball the volume of your favorite foods based on Zone Food Blocks, you'll find making Zone meals by sight alone becomes almost foolproof.

To make it even easier in the first couple of weeks, I recommend using the recipes in my other books to give you an idea what a four-block Zone meal looks like. One note of caution. The only problem with using low-glycemic load carbohydrates like vegetables as your primary source of carbohydrates is that you may have a hard time being able to eat the entire meal. As an example, here is the ingredient list for a four-block meal of Hungarian Chicken, which is typical for a Zone meal.

4 ounces of chicken tenderloin
1 tomato, chopped
2 green and red peppers, cut into strips
¾ cup chopped onions
½ cup chickpeas
1⅓ teaspoons olive oil

Given that this is a serving for one, I'm sure it's not lost on you that given that quantity of vegetables to consume, this may not be an easy meal to finish. This is why your grandmother told you that you couldn't leave the table until you finished your vegetables.

Let's see how these ingredients for Hungarian Chicken can be divided into Zone Food Blocks.

4 ounces of chicken tenderloin = 4 Protein Blocks
and 2 Fat Blocks
1 tomato, chopped = ½ Carbohydrate Block
2 green and red peppers, cut into strips = 1 Carbohydrate
Block
¾ cup chopped onions = ½ Carbohydrate Block
½ cup chickpeas = 2 Carbohydrate Blocks
1⅓ teaspoons olive oil = 2 Fat Blocks

If you add up all of the Zone Food Blocks, here is what you get:

Protein = 4 Blocks
Carbohydrate = 4 Blocks
Fat = 4 Blocks

In other words, it's a balanced Zone meal. More importantly, because Zone Food Blocks are interchangeable, you have the ability to make an infinite number of meals using the foods you like to eat. Just make the corresponding change of one Zone Food Block with another Zone Food Block from the same category, and you now have a new meal.

In addition, there are some frozen dinners and fast-food meals that are pretty close to being in the Zone. These will have equal amounts of protein, carbohydrate, and fat blocks. Let's be frank—these won't be the best-tasting meals, but they can be used in a pinch.

And what about fast-food restaurants? Actually fast-food restaurants have been given a bad rap over the years. They do serve protein in defined sizes (although most of it contains a higher fat content). The only trouble is they also serve amazing amounts of carbohydrate at the same time. Knowing when to hold back on the carbohydrates (and if necessary throw out some of them that come with the meal) is the key to eating fast food in the Zone. But there are many examples (like grilled chicken sandwiches without the mayo or chili), which are surprisingly good and very quick Zone meals. As for other menu items, you have to be a little creative. Let me give you two examples using McDonald's. One might buy two of the cheap hamburgers, then throw away one of the buns, put the two hamburger patties together, and surround them with the remaining bun. *Voilà.* It's a little rich in saturated fat, but at least it's quick. A better choice would be to purchase the McGrilled Chicken sandwich and a McDonald's salad. Throw away ¾ of the bun, put the grilled chicken breast on the salad, and use the remaining ¼ of the bun for your carbohydrate. Much less saturated fat, but still not the most appealing Zone meal.

Of course the best fast-food restaurant remains the supermarket salad bar where you can load up on pre-cut fresh fruits and vegetables. Then walk over to the deli section to get some low-fat protein, and walk back to the salad bar to add a dash of oil and vinegar salad dressing for the necessary fat. It's quick, it's healthy, and it's in the Zone.

MAKING ADJUSTMENTS TO YOUR MEALS
USING ZONE FOOD BLOCKS

Another powerful use of the Zone Food Blocks is to help you convert the meals you already like to eat into Zone meals compatible with your own unique biochemistry. In reality most people tend to eat only about 10 meals at home. How many meals do you really eat for breakfast? For most people, it's probably two. How many do you really eat for lunch? About three. And dinner? Maybe five different meals. That's a total of ten meals. And when you go out to eat, it's probably the same. You eat at your favorite restaurants, eating only your favorite meals. It's just human nature. Using the Zone Food Blocks you can make human nature work in your favor.

By using Zone Food Blocks, you are finally in hormonal control of your diet. Each meal becomes a question of which drug you want to prepare to maintain insulin in the Zone for the next four to six hours. If you think that takes all of the enjoyment out of food, let me remind you that the one region of the world where Zone cooking is commonplace is called France. Gourmet French cooking is really very similar to the Zone in the balance of food blocks at each meal. And no one has ever accused the French of not eating well or not enjoying their food. Maybe that's why they have the lowest rate of heart disease in Europe and actually fit into designer clothing.

READING FOOD LABELS

Food labels can be very useful once you convert frozen meals or fast-food meals into Zone Food Blocks. The conversion of a serving size of protein from the typical food label is pretty easy. First, just take the amount of protein and divide by 7 (remember a protein block is 7 grams), then round that number into the most appropriate whole number. As an example, if a serving size contains 7 grams of protein per serving, this means that each serving size contains one protein block. If it contains 10 grams of protein per serving, then divide 10 by 7 to get 1.4 protein blocks. Just round this down to 1 protein block. If the serving size contains 14 grams of protein, then it contains two protein blocks. You don't have to be obsessive about the calculations, just get a rough idea.

Next, divide the total fat content by 3 (3 grams of fat equals one Zone fat block) and then round to the nearest whole number. If you have less than one fat block for every protein block in prepared meals, then you will have to add some extra fat blocks. Just make sure that they are primarily monounsaturated fat because it is generally the easiest fat to add to a meal. Good sources are olive oil, slivered almonds, or guacamole.

Finally, you will have to calculate the carbohydrate blocks. Unfortunately, the food label will have the combination of both insulin-promoting carbohydrate and fiber contained on the total carbohydrate section of the label. Your first task is to subtract the amount of fiber from the total carbohydrate to get the amount of insulin-promoting carbohydrate in a typical serving size. Divide that number by 10 (for some reason dividing by 9 is a difficult process, so just use the number 10) to get the approximate number of carbohydrate blocks. As you did with the protein blocks, just round this number to the nearest whole number.

Now see if the approximate number of protein blocks is equal to the approximate number of carbohydrate blocks and fat blocks in that frozen meal. If so, you have a Zone meal (perhaps not a great tasting Zone meal, but at least a balanced meal). Unfortunately you will probably find that most frozen meals are primarily carbohydrates with small amounts of protein and not enough fat. So to make it a Zone meal you must make some additions. Let me show you a typical example.

Here's the food label of the Weight Watchers Low-fat Ravioli to illustrate these points.

Nutrition Facts

Serving Size 1
Servings 1

Amount Per Serving

Calories 220   Calories from Fat 15

% Daily Value*

Total Fat 2g

    Saturated Fat 0g

Cholesterol 5mg

Sodium 450mg

Potassium   mg

Total Carbohydrate 43g

    Dietary Fiber 4g

    Sugars 10g

Protein 9g

Figure 4. Nutrition label

What a confusing mess. Now let's translate this food label into Zone blocks, starting with the protein first, since the protein content is the core around which every Zone meal is built.

If you divide the protein amount in the stated serving size (9 g) by the amount of protein in one block (7 g), you get approximately one protein block. Now divide the total fat content by 3 to get approximately one fat block. So at least the protein and fat blocks are in the correct ratio.

Finally let's calculate the number of carbohydrate blocks. Although the total carbohydrate content equals 43 grams, we have to subtract out the 4 grams of fiber to get the total amount of insulin-promoting carbohydrate in this serving size which will be 39 grams. Divide this by 10, and you get approximately four blocks of carbohydrate.

So let's look at our meal. This frozen dinner contains one block of protein, one block of fat, and four blocks of carbohydrate. Nowhere near a Zone meal. In fact, this low-fat, high-carbohydrate meal is a surefire way to increase insulin levels.

Now the challenge is to make this hormonal disaster of a meal into a Zone meal. First, you are going to add another three blocks of low-fat protein to it. That could be 3 oz. of sliced chicken breast. These three added protein blocks to the one protein block already contained within the meal gives a total of four blocks of protein. So now you at least have an equal number of protein and carbohydrate blocks, even though all the carbohydrate blocks are high-glycemic load carbohydrates and thus not the best choices.

Finally, we have to increase the fat content to make this a Zone meal. Since it originally contained only one fat block, you have to add another three fat blocks. So that means you have to add just a dash more of fat. You could add 2 teaspoons of olive oil or 3 teaspoons of slivered almonds. This is not a great amount of extra fat, but enough to improve the taste of the meal and give a better hormonal response. Although this frozen dinner is improved hormonally, you probably realize by now that it is easier and cheaper to make a Zone meal yourself in your own kitchen.

First, don't be overly obsessive about how many Zone Food Blocks there are in a meal, but do be very observant about what that meal looked like and how you felt four hours after eating it. If after four hours you have good mental focus and have no hunger (both a consequence of maintaining adequate blood sugar levels), then you know that the meal you ate was a Zone meal. You can come back to that same meal in the same proportions in the future and experience the same druglike benefits of insulin control.

But what if you are hungry less than four hours after eating a meal? Obviously it wasn't a Zone meal. But with some simple adjustments using the Zone Food Blocks you can make it so. Before you make those adjustments you have to ask yourself one other question: Did you feel loopy after the meal or did you have good mental acuity? If you were unable to concentrate (i.e. loopy) or had a hard time staying awake after the meal, this means that the meal you ate four hours earlier had too many carbohydrate blocks for the number of protein blocks in the same meal. This imbalance of carbohydrate to protein blocks had increased insulin levels, and that resulted in reduced blood sugar levels and the corresponding mental fog. Here's the simple adjustment: make the same meal again keeping the same number of protein blocks but decrease the carbohydrate blocks by one. What you are doing is adjusting your hormonal carburetor, which is controlled by the ratio of protein to carbohydrate blocks in a meal.

On the other hand, if you were hungry four hours after a meal, but had good mental acuity, this means you pushed insulin too low with your previous meal. Your adjustment? Maintain the same amount of protein blocks but increase the carbohydrate blocks by one and have the same meal again in a few days. These simple rules are summarized in Figure 5.

By using Zone Food Blocks, it becomes very easy to make every meal you eat, both inside and outside your home, hormonally correct.

ZONE COMMANDMENTS

Here are the basic Zone commandments. Not only are they easy to remember, but, more importantly, they are easy to follow.

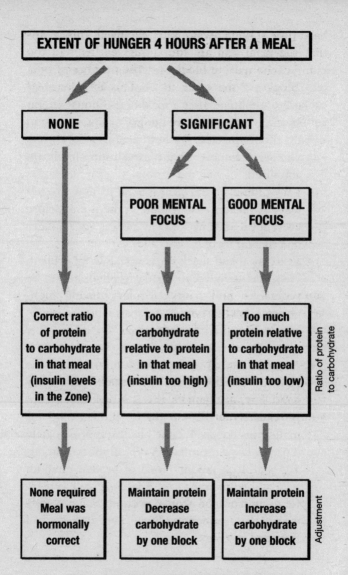

Figure 5. Hormonal Adjustment Diagnostic

- Always eat a Zone meal or snack within one hour after waking
- A Zone meal should give you 4-6 hours in the Zone, a Zone snack 2-3 hours. You must eat every 4-6 hours after a meal or 2-3 hours after a snack, whether you are hungry or not, to stay in the Zone. In fact, the best time to eat is when you aren't hungry. That means insulin levels are stabilized.
- Lack of hunger and clear mental focus are excellent barometers that you are in the Zone. Before every meal and snack always assess your hunger and mental focus.
- Every meal and snack starts with low-fat protein. Next add low-glycemic load carbohydrates (more vegetables and fruits), while reducing high-glycemic load carbohydrates (pasta, breads, grains and starches). Finally add some "good" fats (i.e. olive oil).
- A typical serving size of low-fat protein fits in the palm of your hand and is no thicker than your hand. For most females, this is 3 Zone blocks (approximately 3 oz.) of low-fat protein, and for males, this equals 4 Zone blocks (approximately 4 oz.) of low-fat protein. A typical snack contains 1 Zone block (about 1 oz.) of protein for both men and women. At first, a kitchen scale is helpful to measure the protein portion. You can soon eyeball these amounts at home, in restaurants and fast food takeouts.

- When it comes to low-glycemic load carbohydrates, there really is no need to measure, since it's very difficult to over-consume vegetables and fruits. Simply divide your plate in three equal sections. Add the protein portion and fill the remaining two-thirds of the plate with low-glycemic load vegetables and fruits. Don't forget to add a small amount of fat, like olive oil. If you'd like, include a small salad at dinnertime (a great place to add some "good" fat like olive oil).
- Drink eight 8-ounce glasses of water a day.
- Zone living is guilt free. If you make a mistake don't beat yourself up, your next Zone meal or snack will take you right back to the Zone.
- If all else fails, read *A Week in the Zone*. This is basically the Zone for dummies. Learn to use the eyeball method described in that book, and use the recipes like prescription drugs until you get the hang of the program. But continue to use this book as your reference guide for the Zone Food Blocks.

Once you master the use of Zone Food Blocks, making Zone meals becomes second nature.

THE ZONE FOOD PYRAMID

If you follow these simple instructions, you end with the Zone Food Pyramid.

In fact the pyramid looks suspiciously like the Mediterranean diet since you are eating a lot of vegetables and fruits, adequate amounts of low-fat protein (like fish and chicken), and always adding monounsaturated fat (like olive oil) to every meal. The only difference is that you aren't eating as many high-glycemic load carbohydrates. It is these high-glycemic load carbohydrates that make you fatter and induce more silent inflammation. This is why I tell people the Zone Diet is really the evolution of the Mediterranean diet in that you maintain all of its health benefits without the overproduction of insulin.

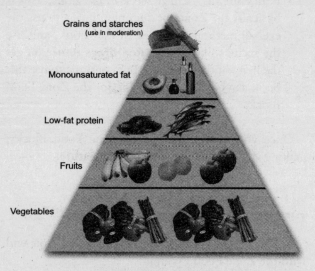

Figure 6. Zone Pyramid

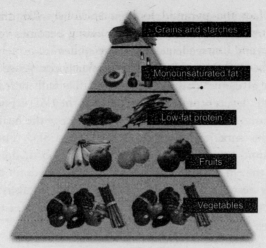

Zone Food Pyramid

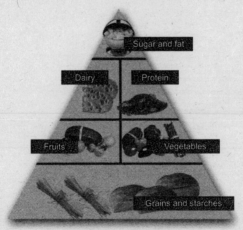

USDA Food Pyramid

**Figure 7. Zone Food Pyramid versus
U.S. Government Food Pyramid**

When you compare the Zone Food Pyramid to the USDA Food Pyramid (shown below) it becomes very apparent why we have an obesity epidemic.

The USDA Food Pyramid is primarily composed of high glycemic load carbohydrates that will increase insulin levels rapidly. It's almost as if the USDA Food Pyramid was launched as a plot to destroy the health of the American people. In fact, the USDA Food Pyramid has done a remarkably good job of doing just that in a little more than a decade. But don't despair because you can reverse this hormonal disaster in less than seven days once you learn to master the Zone.

PART II
The Top Zone Food Ingredients

In my book *The Top 100 Zone Foods,* I described a ranking system to quantify different Zone food ingredients depending on their glycemic load, vitamin and mineral content, levels of anti-oxidants, and monounsaturated fat content. The food ingredients listed in this section are the primary food ingredients you want to use in making Zone meals. To make a perfect Zone meal just make sure all the Zone blocks balance one another in the meal. The typical female will need 3 Zone blocks each of protein, carbohydrate, and fat at every meal, whereas the typical male will need four Zone blocks each of carbohydrate, protein, and fat at every meal. A typical Zone snack consists of one Zone block each of carbohydrate, protein, and fat. You should plan to eat two Zone snacks (one in the late afternoon and one before bedtime) each day.

With a little practice you will quickly find out that the protein will usually occupy one-third of the plate, low-glycemic load carbohydrates take up the other two-thirds, and you will be adding a dash of fat just like I explained using the hand-eye method.

Furthermore, all of the top carbohydrate choices have a low glycemic load if you use the Zone Food Block method. This means by using these carbohydrate ingredients you will significantly reduce the likelihood of type 2 diabetes, heart disease, and silent inflammation. Finally, notice that if you ate only the good (as opposed to very good or best) choices of Zone food ingredients and maintained the right balance of Zone Food Blocks, you would still have highly nutritious meals that any dietician would love. Just think of the nutrition if you used the best Zone ingredients at most of your meals.

TOP CARBOHYDRATE CHOICES

Best Choices	Amount for 1 Zone Block
Blackberries	¾ cup
Blueberries	½ cup
Boysenberries	½ cup
Broccoli (cooked)	3 cups
Broccoli (raw)	4 cups
Cauliflower (raw or cooked)	4 cups
Kale (cooked)	2 cups
Raspberries	1 cup
Romaine lettuce (shredded)	10 cups
Spinach (cooked)	3 cups
Strawberries (finely diced)	1 cup
Swiss chard (cooked)	2½ cups

Very Good Choices

Apricots	3
Artichoke	4 large
Artichoke hearts	1 cup
Asparagus	12 spears
Barley (dry)	½ tablespoon
Beans, black	¼ cup
Beans, green or wax (cooked)	1½ cups
Beans, green (raw)	2 cups
Bok choy (cooked)	3 cups
Brussels sprouts (cooked)	1½ cups
Cabbage (boiled)	3 cups
Cabbage (shredded)	4 cups
Eggplant	1½ cups
Kiwi	1
Lentils (boiled)	¼ cup
Lettuce, iceberg	2 heads
Okra (sliced)	1 cup
Oatmeal, dry (slow cooking)	½ oz.
Oatmeal, cooked (slow cooking)	⅓ cup
Peppers, raw (red or green)	2
Pink grapefruit	½
Plum	1
Tomato, raw	2
Tomato, raw (chopped)	1½ cups
Tomato, cherry (raw)	2 cups
Tomato (canned and chopped)	1 cup
Tomato (puree)	½ cup
Tomato sauce	½ cup
Snow peas, raw	1½ cups

Good Choices

Apple (medium)	½
Applesauce (unsweetened)	⅓ cup

Good Choices (cont'd)

Beans, kidney (boiled)	¼ cup
Cherries	8
Celery, raw (sliced)	2 cups
Chickpeas (raw or boiled)	¼ cup
Cucumber (medium)	1½
Leeks (boiled)	1 cup
Mushrooms (boiled)	2 cups
Mushrooms (raw)	4 cups
Grapes (red or green)	½ cup
Peach	1
Pear	½
Onions (chopped and boiled)	½ cup
Onion, raw (chopped)	1 cup
Orange	½
Orange, mandarin	⅓ cup
Scallions, raw	3 cups
Shallots, raw (diced)	1½ cups
Squash, yellow (boiled)	2 cups
String beans (boiled)	1 cup
Zucchini (boiled)	2 cups

TOP PROTEIN CHOICES

Best Choices	Amount for 1 Zone Block
Crabmeat	1½ oz.
Chicken (hormone-free)	1½ oz.
Cod	1½ oz.
Egg substitutes	¼ cup
Egg whites	2 eggs
Haddock	1½ oz.
Halibut	1½ oz.
Lobster	1½ oz.
Mackerel	1½ oz.
Salmon	1½ oz.

Sardines	1½ oz.
Scallops	1½ oz.
Sea bass	1½ oz.
Shrimp	1½ oz.
Snapper	1½ oz.
Soybean hamburger crumbles	½ cup
Tuna (steak)	1½ oz.
Turkey breast (fresh)	1 oz.

Very Good Choices

Beef (hormone-free)	1 oz.
Chicken breast (fresh)	1 oz.
Cottage cheese (1% fat)	¼ cup
Emu	1 oz.
Freshwater bass	1½ oz.
Soy Canadian bacon	3 slices
Tofu (extra-firm)	2 oz.
Trout	1½ oz.

Good Choices

Beef tenderloin (well-trimmed)	1 oz.
Buffalo	1 oz.
Canadian bacon (lean)	1 oz.
Chicken breast (deli)	1½ oz.
Low-fat cheese	1 oz.
Pork tenderloin (well-trimmed)	1 oz.
Ostrich	1 oz.
Soybean sausage	1 link
Soybean hot dog	1 link
Tuna (canned)	1 oz.
Turkey breast (deli)	1½ oz.
Venison	1 oz.

TOP MIXED PROTEIN SOURCES*

Best Choices	Amount for 1 Zone Block	Associated Carb Blocks
Milk, 1% or skim	1 cup	1 cup
Yogurt, 1% or skim	½ cup	½ cup

Very Good Choices

Soybean hamburger	⅔ patty	⅓
Tempeh	1½ oz.	1
Tofu (soft)	4 oz.	⅓

Good Choices

Soybeans (boiled)	⅓ cup	⅔

TOP FAT CHOICES

Best Choices	Amount for 1 Zone Block
Olive oil	⅔ teaspoon
Olives	5
Macadamia nuts	2

Very Good Choices

Avocado	2 tablespoons
Almond butter	1 teaspoon
Almonds	6
Guacamole	2 tablespoons
Pistachios	6

Good Choices

Cashews	6
Peanuts	6
Canola oil	⅔ teaspoon

---

*These also contain carbohydrates, so read the labels carefully.

Where are you going to find all of these Zone food ingredients? On the periphery of the supermarket. It's within the aisles of the supermarket that all the danger lurks. Here is where the major food companies have spent billions of dollars learning how to stuff starchy carbohydrates and grains into brightly packaged foods that last forever. Unfortunately, these are the same carbohydrates that drive up insulin levels that make you fat and keep you fat. This is not to say you can never have bread, pasta, or rice again, just if you do, use them as condiments, not the major source of carbohydrates on your plate.

One last comment about shopping for Zone meal ingredients. Frozen fruits and vegetables are your best all-around choices economically. They actually have a greater amounts of vitamins than "fresh" fruit and vegetables. This is because frozen fruits and vegetables are frozen immediately after harvest, whereas "fresh" fruits and vegetables have a very long journey from the fields to the distribution center to the supermarket and finally to your refrigerator. More importantly, frozen fruits and vegetables are much better tasting than ever before.

Nonetheless, here are a few hints to make frozen vegetables and fruits taste even better.

1. Place frozen vegetables into an aluminum tent with some olive oil and then sprinkle some lemon juice on them. Heat them in a 450°F oven for 18–20 minutes and then serve.

2. Alternatively, sauté thawed vegetables using refined olive oil. (The heat would destroy the active ingredients in extra virgin olive oil.)

3. Another approach is to grill the vegetables for 10–12 minutes, but don't forget to use olive oil to baste them.

4. Finally you can make a heart-healthy Hollandaise or Béarnaise sauce for the vegetables by replacing butter with olive oil, or simply add a dash of extra virgin olive oil over the vegetables no matter how they are prepared.

5. Finally for frozen fruits, don't be averse to adding a small amount of whipped cream to them. Somehow this makes any fruit taste a lot better.

EATING IN: YOUR HOME ZONE

Surprisingly, most people only eat about 20 different food items. If you doubt me, just make a list. In fact, ask yourself how many of the Top Zone foods appear on that list. Chances are, you need to expand your culinary repertoire. Of course you can still eat your favorite protein, carbohydrate, and fat choices. Just add some new foods to the pot.

As you make your supermarket shopping list each week, make a point of including one or two new foods from my Top Zone Food list that you don't normally buy. Whether it's spinach to mix into your salad, asparagus to add to your omelet, or tofu to mix into your stir-fry vegetables, continually try new combinations. The recipes in this book are just suggestions. You can substitute different kinds of greens in your salads or steamed bok choy instead of broccoli. Whatever works for you.

Most people find it's easy to get stuck in a meal rut, preparing the same meals over and over again, week after week. It's easy, mindless, and less trouble than poring through new recipes. Still, I urge you to try a new food or two every week—or even every day if you can swing it. Just as you can make minor adjustments to your favorite meals to make them Zone-friendly, you can also make a few changes to your Zone meals to get the highest-quality foods. Within a few weeks, you'll have a formidable pharmacy of "drugs" to pick and choose from that will dramatically improve the quality of your life.

YOUR GUIDE TO SUPERMARKET SHOPPING

Your supermarket shopping habits can make or break your commitment to the Zone. Stock your kitchen with the wrong kinds of foods, and you'll be left with no other choice but to eat them when the chips are down and you're famished. Your best bet? Leave the low-quality protein, carbohydrates, and fats where they should be: in someone else's kitchen.

Follow these steps to becoming a savvy supermarket shopper.

Step #1: Always go with a list. Go prepared with a list of high-quality Zone foods, and stick with that list. To help you stick with the list, make sure you don't shop when you're hungry. Eat a Zone meal or snack before you hit the supermarket.

Step #2: Stay mainly on the periphery. Ever notice that the fruits, vegetables, meat, fish, and dairy products are all found in the outer aisles? This is where you want to spend most of your time. Avoid the center aisles, which contain the processed foods like cereals, pasta, and snack foods. And of course, avoid the bakery at all costs.

PART III
Putting It All Together

Making Zone meals is not exactly rocket science. In fact, it's pretty simple. Just remember that each Zone meal must contain protein, carbohydrate and fat, and you must select the same total number of blocks from each group to make a Zone meal. If you are the typical female, make sure that each meal has three (3) choices from each group (i.e., 3 proteins, 3 carbohydrates, and 3 fats). For example, if you select skinless, chicken breast from the protein group, simply triple the Zone Food Block measurement. The actual portion size would be 3 ounces (3 × 1 oz.). Do the same for the carbohydrate and fat portions. Or you may mix items within each group as long as the total number of items selected equals three Zone Carbohydrate blocks (3). For your carbohydrate portion you might select 12 spears of asparagus (1 Block) and 1 cup of blueberries (2 Blocks) for a total of three Blocks. If you are a typical male, have each meal containing four items from each group. Hundreds of Zone meals can be found in my books

Mastering the Zone, Zone Perfect Meals in Minutes, The Soy Zone, and *Zone Meals in Seconds.*

BASIC ZONE RULES

Here are some basic Zone rules to remember:

1. Always eat within 1 hour after waking.
2. Never let more than 5 hours go by without eating a Zone meal or snack whether you are hungry or not.
3. Have some protein at every meal and snack.
4. Eat more fruits and vegetables, and ease off on the bread, pasta, grains, and starches.
5. Make sure you always eat your late afternoon and late evening Zone snacks.
6. Drink at least 64 oz. of liquid (water is the best choice) every day.
7. If you make a mistake, don't worry about it. Just make your next meal a Zone meal.
8. Eat a Zone snack 30 minutes before exercise.

RECIPES FOR A WEEK IN THE ZONE

I want to show you what a typical week in the Zone looks like for both males and females. Each of these meals has the right balance of protein, carbohydrate, and fat, which means that each of these meals can be used like a drug to keep insulin within the Zone for the next four to six hours. More important, they're delicious, and quick and easy to prepare.

If you follow the simple (and great-tasting) meal planner outlined in the following pages, you'll have a surefire path straight into the Zone. Within one week, you'll be looking better, feeling better, and starting your body on a lifelong journey to optimum health by controlling silent inflammation.

7 DAYS IN THE ZONE (FEMALE)
DAY 1

Breakfast: Fruit Salad

Ingredients
- ¾ cup low-fat cottage cheese
- 1 cup fresh or reduced-sugar canned pineapple, cubed
- ⅓ cup reduced-sugar canned mandarin oranges, drained
- 3 macadamia nuts, crushed

Instructions: Place cottage cheese in a bowl. Fold in pineapple, oranges, and nuts.

Lunch: Chef's Salad

Ingredients
- 1 cup green-leaf lettuce (substitute lettuce of your choice), washed, dried, and torn into large pieces

¼ cup canned chickpeas, drained and rinsed

½ cup button mushrooms, washed, dried, and
   coarsely chopped

½ cup celery, washed, dried, and coarsely chopped

1 tablespoon olive oil-and-vinegar dressing*

1½ ounces deli-style turkey breast, cut into strips

1½ ounces deli-style ham, cut into strips

1 ounce reduced-fat Swiss cheese (substitute any
   reduced-fat cheese), julienned

For Dessert
   1 medium apple

Instructions: Toss lettuce with chickpeas, mushrooms, and celery. Dress, toss, and add meat and cheese. Serve apple for dessert.

Late Afternoon: Zone Snack (see page 88)

Dinner: Ginger Chicken

Ingredients
   1 teaspoon olive oil
   3 ounces boneless, skinless chicken breast, cut
      lengthwise into thin strips

---

*Zone oil-and-vinegar dressing contains 1 teaspoon olive oil and 2 teaspoons vinegar. Extra vinegar may be added to taste.

2 cups broccoli florets, washed

1½ cups snow peas, washed

¾ cup yellow onion, peeled and chopped

1 teaspoon fresh ginger, grated

For Dessert

½ cup seedless grapes

Instructions: In a wok or large nonstick pan, heat oil over medium high heat. Add chicken and sauté, turning frequently, until lightly browned, about 5 minutes. Add broccoli, snow peas, onion, ginger, and ¼ cup water. Continue cooking, stirring often, until the chicken is done, water is reduced to a glaze, and vegetables are tender, about 20 minutes. If the pan dries out during cooking, add water in tablespoon increments to keep moist. Serve grapes for dessert.

Late Evening: Zone Snack (see page 88)

DAY 2

Breakfast: Yogurt and Fruit

Ingredients

1 ounce lean Canadian bacon (substitute 3 turkey bacon strips or 2 soy sausage links)

½ cup fresh blueberries, rinsed and drained

1 tablespoon slivered almonds

1 cup plain low-fat yogurt

Instructions: Prepare bacon or soy patties, following package instructions. Stir fruit and nuts into yogurt, and serve with bacon or links on the side.

Lunch: Tuna Salad

Ingredients
   3 ounces albacore tuna packed in water, drained
   ¼ cup celery, washed, dried, and coarsely chopped
   1 tablespoon olive oil-and-vinegar dressing*
   1 or 2 lettuce leaves, washed and dried
   ½ cantaloupe, seeds scooped out
   ½ cup blueberries, rinsed and drained

Instructions: Mix tuna with celery and stir in dressing. Prepare a bed of the lettuce leaves and top with tuna mixture. Stuff cantaloupe with berries and serve for dessert.

Late Afternoon: Zone Snack (see page 88)

Dinner: Foiled Flounder with Green Beans

Ingredients
   vegetable spray
   4½ ounces boneless flounder fillet (substitute mild, flaky fish of your choice)

---

*Zone oil-and-vinegar dressing contains 1 teaspoon olive oil and 2 teaspoons vinegar. Extra vinegar may be added to taste.

2 tablespoons yellow onion, peeled and chopped
sprinkling of Parmesan cheese
¼ teaspoon freshly ground pepper, or to taste
squirt lemon juice
1½ cups fresh green beans, washed, ends removed,
    and halved
1 tablespoon almonds, slivered

For Dessert
½ cup of fresh or frozen blueberries

Instructions: Preheat oven to 425°. Tear off an 18-
by-12-inch piece of foil. Spray the center lightly
with vegetable spray, and place fish in the center of
the foil. Top with onion and sprinkle with cheese,
pepper, and lemon juice. Fold foil loosely over fish,
leaving ample space for air. Carefully turn up and
seal the ends and the middle so that juices won't
leak out. Bake in the preheated oven 18 minutes.
Meanwhile, steam the green beans: in a large pot fitted with a steaming basket, bring 1 inch water to
boil. Add beans to the basket and steam until crisp-
tender, 10 minutes. Drain, place in serving bowl,
and fold in almonds. When fish is done, carefully
open foil to prevent steam burns, and remove to a
plate. Serve with green beans. Serve pineapple for
dessert.

Late Evening: Zone Snack (see page 88)

DAY 3

Breakfast: Fruit Smoothie

Ingredients

20 grams protein powder
1 cup blueberries
1 cup strawberries
3 macadamia nuts
4 ice cubes

Instructions: Place all ingredients in a blender and blend at high speed until smooth, about 1 minute. Add a little water if smoothie is too thick. If you prefer, eat the nuts on the side.

Lunch: Cheeseburger

Ingredients

3 ounces lean (less than 10% fat) ground beef (substitute 3 ounces ground turkey or 1 soy burger patty)
1 ounce reduced-fat American cheese (substitute cheese of choice)
1 tablespoon light mayonnaise
½ hamburger roll
1 thick tomato slice, optional
1 large lettuce leaf, optional
1 dill pickle wedge, optional

For Dessert
⅔ cup unsweetened applesauce
sprinkling of cinnamon

Instructions: Preheat broiler. Place burger on foil or rack and broil 5 minutes. Flip and continue cooking another 5 minutes for medium rare. One minute before expected doneness, top with cheese, and remove when melted. Spread mayonnaise on the roll. Top with burger, tomato, and lettuce. Serve pickle on the side. Sprinkle applesauce with cinnamon and serve for dessert.

Late Afternoon: Zone Snack (see page 88)

Dinner: Vegetarian Stir-fry

Ingredients
1 teaspoon olive oil
⅔ cup vegetable protein crumbles* (substitute 4 ounces firm tofu)
1½ cups yellow onions, peeled and chopped
2 cups broccoli florets, washed
2 cups button mushrooms, washed, dried, and thinly sliced

---

*Morningstar Farms makes Burger-Style Recipe Crumbles, which looks like ground beef and is a good vegetarian source of protein.

---

1 ounce reduced-fat Swiss cheese,
   shredded

For Dessert
   ½ cup grapes

Instructions: Heat oil in a nonstick sauté pan or wok over medium-high heat. If using tofu, remove from wrapping, drain, and crumble. Add tofu or soy crumbles and stir until mixed with the oil. Add onions, broccoli, and mushrooms. Reduce heat to medium and stir-fry, stirring often, until vegetables are tender, about 15 minutes. Stir in cheese and heat until melted, about 1 minute. Serve grapes for dessert.

Late Evening: Zone Snack (see page 88)

DAY 4

Breakfast: Scrambled Eggs and Bacon

Ingredients
   vegetable spray
   4 egg whites (or ½ cup egg substitute)
   1 teaspoon olive oil
   1 tablespoon low-fat milk (optional)
   1 ounce lean Canadian bacon (substitute 3 turkey
      bacon strips or 2 soy sausage links)

For Dessert
    1 cup grapes
    ⅓ cup Mandarin oranges

Instructions: Lightly coat a large nonstick pan with vegetable spray, and heat over medium flame. Beat egg whites with olive oil and milk, if desired. Pour into pan and cook, stirring often, until scrambled and fully set. Prepare bacon or soy links, following package instructions. Mix grapes and oranges and serve for dessert.

Lunch: Tofu Dip and Veggies

Ingredients
    4 ounces firm tofu
    1 ounce reduced-fat Swiss cheese, grated
    ¼ cup canned chickpeas, drained and rinsed
    1 teaspoon olive oil
    2 tablespoons fresh lemon juice
    2 tablespoons Lipton's dry onion soup mix (substitute
        spices of your choice, to taste*)
    1 medium green pepper, washed, cored, seeded, and
        cut in wedges
    2 cups broccoli florets

*If you don't want to use the packaged soup mix, experiment with minced onions, garlic, or vegetable bouillon granules.

For Dessert
    Kiwi

Instructions: Drain tofu. Put tofu, cheese, chickpeas, olive oil, lemon juice, and onion soup mix in a blender. Blend until smooth. (For best flavor, refrigerate the dip at least 2 hours or overnight.) Place dip in a bowl in the center of a large plate. Arrange pepper strips and broccoli around bowl for dipping. Serve kiwi for dessert.

Late Afternoon: Zone Snack (see page 88)

Dinner: Spiced Lamb with Vegetables

Ingredients
    4½ ounces lean ground lamb
    1 teaspoon cider vinegar
    1 teaspoon olive oil
    ½ cup scallions, finely chopped
    ¾ cup red onions, cut in chunks
    2 cups mushrooms
    1½ cups tomatoes, diced
    ½ cup green beans, diced
    1 tablespoon cilantro
    2 teaspoons fresh ginger, minced
    ¼ teaspoon cumin
    ¼ teaspoon coriander
    ⅛ teaspoon black pepper

½ teaspoon celery salt
⅛ teaspoon cinnamon

Instructions: In a small glass bowl, combine lamb, vinegar, and spices. Cover and refrigerate for 30 minutes. Heat the oil in a medium nonstick sauté pan. Add meat mixture and vegetables. Cook, breaking meat up as it cooks, until lamb is cooked through and vegetables are tender. Spoon onto plate and serve.

Late Evening: Zone Snack (see page 88)

DAY 5

Breakfast: Old-fashioned Oatmeal

Ingredients
⅔ cup slow-cooking (steel-cut) oatmeal*
2 ounces lean Canadian bacon (substitute 6 turkey bacon strips or 2 soy sausage links)
⅓ cup unsweetened applesauce
1 tablespoon almonds, slivered
sprinkling of nutmeg
sprinkling of cinnamon
¼ cup low-fat cottage cheese

---

*By slow cooking, I mean slow cooking. Oatmeal that calls itself slow-cooking but takes only 5 minutes isn't the real McCoy (or perhaps I should say the real McCann's, a popular brand). To shorten the morning cooking time, make a big batch during the weekend, freeze, and microwave the correct amount in the morning. You may also put the oatmeal in a wide-mouth thermos with 1⅓ cups boiling water, and let it cook overnight.

Instructions: Bring 3 cups water to a brisk boil over high heat. Add oatmeal, stirring well. When smooth and beginning to thicken, reduce heat to low and simmer for 30 minutes, stirring occasionally. While oatmeal is cooking, prepare bacon or soy patties, following package instructions. Remove oatmeal from the heat. Stir in applesauce and almonds. Sprinkle with cinnamon and nutmeg. Serve bacon and cottage cheese on the side.

Lunch: Chili (Meat or Vegetarian)

Ingredients
   1 teaspoon olive oil
   4½ ounces lean (less than 10%) ground beef
      (substitute ground turkey or 1 cup vegetable
      protein crumbles*)
   ¼ cup yellow onions, peeled and minced
   1 teaspoon chili powder, or to taste
   ½ teaspoon garlic powder, or to taste
   ½ teaspoon freshly ground pepper, or to taste
   1 cup salsa or stewed tomatoes with liquid
   ¼ cup kidney beans, drained and rinsed
   Sprinkling of low-fat Monterey Jack cheese (optional)

Instructions: In a large nonstick sauté pan, heat oil over medium-high flame. Add meat and sauté, stirring

---

*Morningstar Farms makes Burger Style Recipe Crumbles, which looks like ground beef and is a good vegetarian source of protein.

often, until lightly browned, about 5 minutes. If using protein crumbles, heat until blended with oil, about 2 minutes. Add onions, chili powder, garlic powder, pepper, salsa, and kidney beans. Simmer, stirring occasionally, until onion is wilted and flavors are blended, about 20 minutes. Place in bowl and top with cheese, if desired.

Late Afternoon: Zone Snack (see page 88)

Dinner: Shrimp Scampi with Vegetables

Ingredients

1 teaspoon olive oil

1 cup asparagus spears, washed, woody bases discarded, and bias-sliced into 1-inch-long pieces

¾ cup yellow onions, peeled and finely chopped

1 medium green pepper, washed, cored, seeded, and roughly chopped

2 cloves garlic, peeled and minced, or to taste

4½ ounces shrimp, shelled and deveined

¼ cup dry white wine (optional)

1–2 teaspoons lemon juice, or to taste

2 lemon wedges, optional

For Dessert

1 medium peach

Instructions: In a large nonstick pan, heat oil over medium-high heat. Sauté asparagus, onions, green pepper, and garlic, stirring often until tender, about 10 minutes. Add shrimp, white wine, and lemon juice. Lower heat to medium and cook 5 minutes, stirring often, until shrimp are pink. Place on plate and garnish with lemon wedges. Serve peach for dessert.

Late Evening: Zone Snack (see page 88)

DAY 6

Breakfast: Spanish Omelet

Ingredients

vegetable spray

2 tablespoons yellow onion, peeled and finely chopped*

2 tablespoons green pepper, cored, seeded, and roughly chopped*

4 large egg whites (or ½ cup egg substitute)

1 tablespoon low-fat milk (optional)

1 teaspoon chili powder, or to taste (optional)

1 teaspoon olive oil

¼ cup canned black beans, drained

---

*No one wants to chop vegetables first thing in the morning. Buy a bag of frozen onions and green peppers and just pour out what you need. Return the rest to the freezer.

---

1 ounce low-fat Monterey Jack cheese, shredded
1 tablespoon salsa (optional)

For Dessert
1 medium orange

Instructions: Lightly coat a large nonstick sauté pan with vegetable spray, and heat over medium flame. Add onion and green pepper and sauté, stirring often, until tender, about 10 minutes. Remove and set aside. Meanwhile, beat egg whites with milk, if desired. Stir in chili powder. Heat olive oil in the large nonstick sauté pan over medium heat. Pour in the egg whites and cook until almost set, occasionally lifting edges so that uncooked portion flows underneath, 2 to 3 minutes. When eggs are set, place onions, green pepper, black beans, and cheese on top. Fold with a spatula and continue cooking until lightly browned, about 1 minute. Top with salsa. Serve orange for dessert.

Lunch: Grilled Chicken Salad

Ingredients
1 cup green-leaf or romaine lettuce, washed, dried, and torn into large pieces
1 cup broccoli florets
½ green pepper, cored, seeded, and cut into thin strips
1 medium tomato, sliced

1 tablespoon olive-oil-and-vinegar dressing*
1 tablespoon lemon juice
1 teapoon Worcestershire sauce
½ teaspoon freshly ground pepper, or to taste
4 ounces precooked grilled skinless chicken breast,
   sliced into bite-sized chunks

For Dessert
1 medium pear

Instructions: Toss lettuce with broccoli, green pepper, kidney beans, and tomato. Combine dressing with the lemon juice, Worcestershire sauce, and pepper. Toss with vegetables until well combined, and top with chicken chunks. Serve pear for dessert.

Late afternoon: Zone snack (see page 88)

Dinner: Broiled Salmon

Ingredients
6 ounces salmon steak, about 1 inch thick
1 ⅓ teaspoons olive oil
½ teaspoon dried rosemary, or to taste
½ teaspoon dried tarragon, or to taste
½ teaspoon dried dill, or to taste
2 cups zucchini, washed, ends removed, and sliced
   into ¼-inch strips

---

*Zone oil-and-vinegar dressing contains 1 teaspoon olive oil and 2 teaspoons vinegar. Extra vinegar may be added to taste.

For Dessert
    1 apple
    1 plum

Instructions: Preheat broiler. Brush salmon with olive oil and sprinkle with herbs. On a roasting pan or aluminum foil, broil for 4–5 minutes per side, depending on thickness, turning once. Meanwhile, steam the zucchini: in a large pot fitted with a steaming basket, bring 1 inch water to boil. Add zucchini to the basket and steam until crisp-tender, 4 to 6 minutes. Serve apple and plum for dessert.

Late evening: Zone snack (see page 88)

DAY 7

Breakfast: Vegetable Omelet

Ingredients
    1 cup asparagus spears, woody bases discarded,
        bias-sliced into 1-inch pieces
    1 ⅓ teaspoons olive oil
    ¼ cup yellow onions, peeled and finely chopped
    ½ cup button mushrooms, washed, dried,
        and thinly sliced
    6 egg whites (or ¾ cup egg substitute)
    1 tablespoon low-fat milk (optional)
    vegetable spray
    3 strips turkey bacon (substitute 1 ounce lean
        Canadian bacon or 2 soy sausage links)
    1 cup Mandarin oranges

Instructions: In a large pot fitted with a steaming basket, bring 1 inch water to boil. Add asparagus to the basket and steam until crisp-tender, 5 minutes, and set aside. Heat olive oil in a large nonstick sauté pan over medium heat. Add onions and mushrooms and lightly sauté until onion is wilted, about 10 minutes. Remove from pan and set aside to cool. Meanwhile, beat egg whites with milk, if desired. Stir in cooled onions and mushrooms. Lightly coat the sauté pan with vegetable spray, and heat over medium flame. Pour in the egg mixture and cook until almost set, occasionally lifting edges so that uncooked portion flows underneath, 2 to 3 minutes. When eggs are set, top with asparagus tips and fold with a spatula. Continue cooking until lightly browned, about 1 minute. Prepare bacon or soy links, following package instructions, and serve on the side with oranges.

Lunch: Stuffed Tomatoes

Ingredients
- 3 ounces albacore tuna packed in water, drained
- 1 tablespoon light mayonnaise
- ¼ cup celery, washed and minced
- 1 tablespoon onion, peeled and minced
- 2 large tomatoes, washed, tops removed, and hulled

For Dessert
- 1 nectarine

Instructions: In a medium mixing bowl, combine tuna, mayonnaise, celery, and onion. Stuff into tomatoes and serve. Serve nectarine for dessert.

Late Afternoon: Zone Snack (see page 88)

Dinner: Chicken Marinara with Three-Bean Salad*

Ingredients
    1½ cups green beans, washed, ends removed, and
        cut in half
    ¼ cup canned chickpeas, drained
    ¼ cup canned kidney beans, drained
    1 teaspoon olive oil
    2 tablespoons cider vinegar, or to taste
    1 teaspoon dried chives
    1 teaspoon dried parsley
    ½ teaspoon freshly ground pepper, or to taste
    1½ teaspoons dried basil
    2 ounces boneless, skinless chicken breast cutlets
    2 tablespoons prepared tomato sauce
    ¼ teaspoon garlic powder, or to taste
    1 ounce low-fat mozzarella cheese, shredded

---

*If possible, make three-bean salad ahead of time (up to 2 days) and store, tightly sealed, in the refrigerator.

Instructions: Preheat oven to 450°. In a large pot fitted with a steaming basket, bring 1 inch water to boil. Add green beans to the basket and steam until crisp-tender, 10 minutes. Remove from basket, drain, and combine with chickpeas and kidney beans. In a small mixing bowl, combine olive oil, vinegar, chives, parsley, pepper, and 1 teaspoon of the basil; experiment with the oil-vinegar ratio to taste. Toss with beans, cover, and refrigerate for 30 minutes. Place chicken in a large piece of foil. Top chicken with tomato sauce and sprinkle with the remaining ½ teaspoon basil, garlic powder, and cheese. Fold foil loosely over chicken, leaving ample space for air. Carefully turn up and seal the ends and the middle so that juices won't leak out. Bake in the preheated oven for 20 minutes. Remove from oven and carefully open foil to prevent steam burns. Serve with bean salad.

Late evening: Zone Snack (see page 88)

7 DAYS IN THE ZONE (MALE)
DAY 1

Breakfast: Fruit Salad

Ingredients
    1 cup low-fat cottage cheese
    1 cup fresh or reduced-sugar canned pineapple,
       cubed

⅔ cup reduced-sugar canned Mandarin oranges,
    drained
4 macadamia nuts, crushed

Instructions: Place cottage cheese in a bowl. Fold in
pineapple, oranges, and nuts.

Lunch: Chef's Salad

Ingredients
    1 cup green-leaf lettuce (substitute lettuce of your
        choice), washed, dried, and torn into large pieces
    ½ cup canned chickpeas, drained and rinsed
    ½ cup button mushrooms, washed, dried, and
        coarsely chopped
    ½ cup celery, washed, dried, and coarsely chopped
    4 teaspoons olive oil-and-vinegar dressing*
    3 ounces deli-style turkey breast, cut into strips
    1½ ounces deli-style ham, cut into strips
    1 ounce reduced-fat Swiss cheese (substitute any
        reduced-fat cheese), julienned

For Dessert
    1 medium apple

---

*Zone oil-and-vinegar dressing for this meal contains 1⅓ tea-
spoons olive oil and 2 teaspoons vinegar. Extra vinegar may be
added to taste.

Instructions: Toss lettuce with chickpeas, mushrooms, and celery. Dress, toss, and add meat and cheese. Serve apple for dessert.

Late Afternoon: Zone Snack (see page 88)

Dinner: Ginger Chicken

Ingredients
  1⅓ teaspoons olive oil
  4 ounces boneless, skinless chicken breast, cut
      lengthwise into thin strips
  2 cups broccoli florets, washed
  1½ cups snow peas, washed
  ¾ cup yellow onion, peeled and chopped
  1 teaspoon fresh ginger, grated

For Dessert
  1 cup seedless grapes

Instructions: In a wok or large nonstick pan, heat oil over medium-high heat. Add chicken and sauté, turning frequently, until lightly browned, about 5 minutes. Add broccoli, snow peas, onion, ginger, and ¼ cup water. Continue cooking, stirring often, until the chicken is done, water is reduced to a glaze, and vegetables are tender, about 20 minutes. If the pan dries out during cooking, add water in tablespoon increments to keep moist. Serve grapes for dessert.

Late Evening: Zone Snack (see page 88)

DAY 2

Breakfast: Yogurt and Fruit

Ingredients

- 1 ounce lean Canadian bacon (substitute 3 turkey bacon strips or 2 soy sausage links)
- ½ cup fresh blueberries, rinsed and drained
- 4 teaspoons slivered almonds
- 1½ cups plain low-fat yogurt

Instructions: Prepare bacon or soy patties, following package instructions. Stir fruit and nuts into yogurt, and serve with bacon or links on the side.

Lunch: Tuna Salad

Ingredients

- 4 ounces albacore tuna packed in water, drained
- ¼ cup celery, washed, dried, and coarsely chopped
- 4 teaspoons olive oil-and-vinegar dressing*

---

*Zone oil-and-vinegar dressing for this meal contains 1⅓ teaspoons olive oil and 2 teaspoons vinegar. Extra vinegar may be added to taste.

---

1 or 2 lettuce leaves, washed and dried
½ cantaloupe, seeds scooped out
¾ cup blueberries, rinsed and drained

Instructions: Mix tuna with celery and stir in dressing. Prepare a bed of the lettuce, and top with tuna mixture. Stuff cantaloupe with berries and serve for dessert.

Late Afternoon: Zone Snack (see page 88)

Dinner: Foiled Flounder with Green Beans

Ingredients
    vegetable spray
    6 ounces boneless flounder fillet (substitute mild, flaky fish of your choice)
    2 tablespoons yellow onion, peeled and chopped
    sprinkling of Parmesan cheese
    ¼ teaspoon freshly ground pepper, or to taste
    squirt lemon juice
    3 cups fresh green beans, washed, ends removed, and halved
    4 teaspoons almonds, slivered

For Dessert
    1 cup of fresh or frozen blueberries

Instructions: Preheat oven to 425°. Tear off an 18-inch-by-12-inch piece of foil. Spray the center lightly with vegetable spray, and place fish in the center of the foil. Top with onion and sprinkle with cheese, pepper, and lemon juice. Fold foil loosely over fish, leaving ample space for air. Carefully turn up and seal the ends and the middle so that juices won't leak out. Bake in the preheated oven 18 minutes. Meanwhile, steam the green beans: in a large pot fitted with a steaming basket, bring 1 inch water to boil. Add beans to the basket and steam until crisp-tender, 10 minutes. Drain, place in serving bowl, and fold in almonds. When fish is done, carefully open foil to prevent steam burns, and remove to a plate. Serve with green beans. Serve pineapple for dessert.

Late Evening: Zone Snack (see page 88)

DAY 3

Breakfast: Fruit Smoothie

Ingredients

    27 grams protein powder
    1¼ cup blueberries
    1½ cup strawberries
    4 macadamia nuts
    6 ice cubes

Instructions: Place all ingredients in a blender and blend at high speed until smooth, about 1 minute. Add a little water if smoothie is too thick. If you prefer, eat the nuts on the side.

Lunch: Cheeseburger

Ingredients

4½ ounces lean (less than 10%) ground beef (substitute 4½ ounces ground turkey or 1½ soy burger patties)

1 ounce reduced-fat American cheese (substitute cheese of choice)

1 tablespoon light mayonnaise

½ hamburger roll

1 thick tomato slice, optional

1 large lettuce leaf, optional

1 dill pickle wedge, optional

3 black olives

For Dessert

1 cup unsweetened applesauce

sprinkling of cinnamon

Instructions: Preheat broiler. Place burger on foil or rack and broil 5 minutes. Flip and continue cooking another 5 minutes for medium rare. One minute before expected doneness, top with cheese, and remove when melted. Spread mayonnaise on the roll. Top with burger, tomato, and lettuce. Serve pickle on the side. Either chop olives and place on top of cheese-burger or serve them on the side. Sprinkle applesauce with cinnamon and serve for dessert.

Late Afternoon: Zone Snack (see page 88)

Dinner: Vegetarian Stir-fry

Ingredients

    1⅓ teaspoons olive oil
    1 cup vegetable protein crumbles* (substitute 6
        ounces firm tofu)
    1½ cups yellow onions, peeled and chopped
    2 cups broccoli florets, washed
    2 cups button mushrooms, washed, dried,
        and thinly sliced
    1 ounce reduced-fat Swiss cheese, shredded

For Dessert

    1 cup grapes

Instructions: Heat oil in a nonstick sauté pan or wok over medium-high heat. If using tofu, remove from wrapping, drain, and crumble. Add tofu or soy crumbles and stir until mixed with the oil. Add onions,

---

*Morningstar Farms makes Burger Style Recipe Crumbles, which looks like ground beef and is a good vegetarian source of protein.

broccoli, and mushrooms. Reduce heat to medium and stir-fry, stirring often, until vegetables are tender, about 15 minutes. Stir in cheese and heat until melted, about 1 minute. Serve grapes for dessert.

Late Evening: Zone Snack (see page 88)

DAY 4

Breakfast: Scrambled Eggs and Bacon

Ingredients
    vegetable spray
    6 egg whites (or ¾ cup egg substitute)
    1⅓ teaspoons olive oil
    1 tablespoon low-fat milk (optional)
    1 ounce lean Canadian bacon (substitute 3 turkey
        bacon strips or 2 soy sausage links)

For Dessert
    1 cup grapes
    ⅔ cup Mandarin oranges

Instructions: Lightly coat a large nonstick pan with vegetable spray, and heat over medium flame. Beat egg whites with olive oil and milk, if desired. Pour into pan and cook, stirring often, until scrambled and fully set. Prepare bacon or soy links, following package instructions. Mix grapes and oranges and serve for dessert.

Lunch: Tofu Dip and Veggies

Ingredients
  6 ounces firm tofu
  1 ounce reduced-fat Swiss cheese, grated
  ½ cup canned chickpeas, drained and rinsed
  1⅓ teaspoons olive oil
  2 tablespoons fresh lemon juice
  2 tablespoons Lipton dry onion soup mix (substitute
      spices of your choice, to taste*)
  1 medium green pepper, washed, cored, seeded, and
      cut in wedges
  2 cups broccoli florets

For Dessert
  1 kiwi

Instructions: Drain tofu. Put tofu, cheese, chickpeas, olive oil, lemon juice, and onion soup mix in a blender. Blend until smooth. (For best flavor, refrigerate the dip at least 2 hours or overnight.) Place dip in a bowl in the center of a large plate. Arrange pepper strips and broccoli around bowl for dipping. Serve kiwi for dessert.

Late Afternoon: Zone Snack (see page 88)

---

*If you don't want to use the packaged soup mix, experiment with minced onions, garlic, or vegetable bouillon granules.

Dinner: Spiced Lamb with Vegetables

Ingredients

  6 ounces lean ground lamb
  ⅕ cup brown rice
  1 teaspoon cider vinegar
  1⅓ teaspoons olive oil
  ½ cup scallions, finely chopped
  ¾ cup red onions, cut in chunks
  2 cups mushrooms
  1½ cups tomatoes, diced
  ½ cup green beans, diced
  1 tablespoon cilantro
  2 teaspoons fresh ginger, minced
  ¼ teaspoon cumin
  ¼ teaspoon coriander
  ⅛ teaspoon black pepper
  ½ teaspoon celery salt
  ⅛ teaspoon cinnamon

Instructions: In a small glass bowl, combine lamb, rice, vinegar, and spices. Cover and refrigerate for 30 minutes. Heat the oil in a medium nonstick sauté pan. Add meat mixture and vegetables. Cook, breaking meat up as it cooks, until lamb is cooked through and vegetables are tender. Spoon onto plate and serve.

Late Evening: Zone Snack (see page 88)

DAY 5

Breakfast: Old-Fashioned Oatmeal

Ingredients
    1 cup slow-cooking (steel-cut) oatmeal*
    2 ounces lean Canadian bacon (substitute 6 turkey
        bacon strips or 1 soy sausage patty)
    ⅓ cup unsweetened applesauce
    1 tablespoon almonds, slivered
    sprinkling of nutmeg
    sprinkling of cinnamon
    ½ cup low-fat cottage cheese

Instructions: Bring 3 cups water to a brisk boil over high heat. Add oatmeal, stirring well. When smooth and beginning to thicken, reduce heat to low and simmer for 30 minutes, stirring occasionally. While oatmeal is cooking, prepare bacon or soy patties, following package instructions. Remove oatmeal from the heat. Stir in applesauce and almonds. Sprinkle with cinnamon and nutmeg. Serve bacon and cottage cheese on the side.

---

*By slow cooking, I mean *slow* cooking. Oatmeal that calls itself slow-cooking but takes only 5 minutes isn't the real McCoy (or perhaps I should say the real McCann's, a popular brand). To shorten the morning cooking time, make a big batch during the weekend, freeze, and microwave the correct amount in the morning. You may also put the oatmeal in a wide-mouth thermos with 1⅓ cups boiling water, and let it cook overnight.

Lunch: Chili (Meat or Vegetarian)

Ingredients

1⅓ teaspoons olive oil

6 ounces lean (less than 10%) ground beef
(substitute ground turkey or 1⅓ cups vegetable
protein crumbles*)

¼ cup yellow onions, peeled and minced

1 teaspoon chili powder, or to taste

½ teaspoon garlic powder, or to taste

½ teaspoon freshly ground pepper, or to taste

1½ cups salsa or stewed tomatoes with liquid

¼ cup kidney beans, drained and rinsed

sprinkling of low-fat Monterey Jack cheese (optional)

Instructions: In a large nonstick sauté pan, heat oil over medium-high flame. Add meat and sauté, stirring often, until lightly browned, about 5 minutes. If using protein crumbles, heat until blended with oil, about 2 minutes. Add onions, chili powder, garlic powder, pepper, salsa, and kidney beans. Simmer, stirring occasionally, until onion is wilted and flavors are blended, about 20 minutes. Place in bowl and top with cheese, if desired.

Late Afternoon: Zone Snack (see page 88)

---

*Morningstar Farms makes Burger Style Recipe Crumbles, which looks like ground beef and is a good vegetarian source of protein.

Dinner: Shrimp Scampi with Vegetables

Ingredients
- 1⅓ teaspoons olive oil
- 1½ cups asparagus spears, washed, woody bases discarded, and bias-sliced into 1-inch-long pieces
- 1½ cups yellow onions, peeled and finely chopped
- 1 medium green pepper, washed, cored, seeded, and roughly chopped
- 2 cloves garlic, peeled and minced, or to taste
- 6 ounces shrimp, shelled and deveined
- ¼ cup dry white wine (optional)
- 1–2 teaspoons lemon juice, or to taste
- 2 lemon wedges, optional

For Dessert
- 1 medium peach

Instructions: In a large nonstick pan, heat oil over medium-high heat. Sauté asparagus, onions, green pepper, and garlic, stirring often, until tender, about 10 minutes. Add shrimp, white wine, and lemon juice. Lower heat to medium and cook 5 minutes, stirring often, until shrimp are pink. Place on plate and garnish with lemon wedges. Serve peach for dessert.

Late Evening: Zone Snack (see page 88)

Breakfast: Spanish Omelet

Ingredients
    vegetable spray
    2 tablespoons yellow onion, peeled and finely
        chopped*
    2 tablespoons green pepper, cored, seeded, and
        roughly chopped*
    6 large egg whites (or ¾ cup egg substitute)
    1 tablespoon low-fat milk (optional)
    1 teaspoon chili powder, or to taste (optional)
    1⅓ teaspoons olive oil
    ½ cup canned black beans, drained
    1 ounce low-fat Monterey Jack cheese, shredded
    1 tablespoon salsa (optional)

For Dessert
    1 medium orange

Instructions: Lightly coat a large nonstick sauté pan with vegetable spray, and heat over medium flame. Add onion and green pepper and sauté, stirring often, until tender, about 10 minutes. Remove and set aside. Meanwhile, beat egg whites with milk, if desired. Stir in chili powder. Heat olive oil in the large nonstick sauté pan over medium heat. Pour in the egg

---

*No one wants to chop vegetables first thing in the morning. Buy a bag of frozen onions and green peppers and just pour out what you need. Return the rest to the freezer.

---

whites and cook until almost set, occasionally lifting edges so that uncooked portion flows underneath, 2 to 3 minutes. When eggs are set, place onions, green pepper, black beans, and cheese on top. Fold with a spatula and continue cooking until lightly browned, about 1 minute. Top with salsa. Serve orange for dessert.

Lunch: Grilled Chicken Salad

Ingredients

2 cups green-leaf or romaine lettuce, washed, dried, and torn into large pieces

1 cup broccoli florets

½ green pepper, cored, seeded, and cut into thin strips

¼ cup canned kidney beans, rinsed and drained

1 medium tomato, sliced

4 teaspoons olive oil-and-vinegar dressing*

1 tablespoon lemon juice

1 teaspoon Worcestershire sauce

½ teaspoon freshly ground pepper, or to taste

4 ounces precooked grilled skinless chicken breast, sliced into bite-sized chunks

---

*Zone oil-and-vinegar dressing for this meal contains 1⅓ teaspoons olive oil and 2 teaspoons vinegar. Extra vinegar may be added to taste.

For Dessert
    1 medium pear

Instructions: Toss lettuce with broccoli, green pepper, kidney beans, and tomato. Combine dressing with the lemon juice, Worcestershire sauce, and pepper. Toss with vegetables until well combined, and top with chicken chunks. Serve pear for dessert.

Late Afternoon: Zone Snack (see page 88)

Dinner: Broiled Salmon

Ingredients
    6 ounces salmon steak, about 1 inch thick
    1⅓ teaspoons olive oil
    ½ teaspoon dried rosemary, or to taste
    ½ teaspoon dried tarragon, or to taste
    ½ teaspoon dried dill, or to taste
    2 cups zucchini, washed, ends removed, and sliced
        into ¼-inch strips

For Dessert
    1 apple
    1 plum

Instructions: Preheat broiler. Brush salmon with olive oil and sprinkle with herbs. On a roasting pan or aluminum foil, broil for 4-5 minutes per side, depending on thickness, turning once. Meanwhile, steam the zucchini: in a large pot fitted with a steaming basket, bring 1 inch water to boil. Add zucchini to the basket and steam until crisp-tender, 4 to 6 minutes. Serve apple and plum for dessert.

Late Evening: Zone Snack (see page 88)

DAY 7

Breakfast: Vegetable Omelet

Ingredients
    1 cup asparagus spears, woody bases discarded, bias-sliced into 1-inch pieces
    1⅓ teaspoons olive oil
    ¼ cup yellow onions, peeled and finely chopped
    ½ cup button mushrooms, washed, dried, and thinly sliced
    6 egg whites (or ¾ cup egg substitute)
    1 tablespoon low-fat milk (optional)
    vegetable spray
    3 strips turkey bacon (substitute 1 ounce lean Canadian bacon or 2 soy sausage links)
    1 cup Mandarin oranges

Instructions: In a large pot fitted with a steaming basket, bring 1 inch water to boil. Add asparagus to the basket and steam until crisp-tender, 5 minutes, and set aside. Heat olive oil in a large nonstick sauté pan over medium heat. Add onions and mushrooms and lightly sauté until onion is wilted, about 10 minutes. Remove from pan and set aside to cool. Meanwhile, beat egg whites with milk, if desired. Stir in cooled onions and mushrooms. Lightly coat the sauté pan with vegetable spray, and heat over medium flame. Pour in the egg mixture and cook until almost set, occasionally lifting edges so that uncooked portion flows underneath, 2 to 3 minutes. When eggs are set, top with asparagus tips and fold with a spatula. Continue cooking until lightly browned, about 1 minute. Prepare bacon or soy links, following package instructions, and serve on the side with oranges.

Lunch: Stuffed Tomatoes

Ingredients
    4 ounces albacore tuna packed in water, drained
    4 teaspoons light mayonnaise
    ¼ cup celery, washed and minced
    1 tablespoon onion, peeled and minced
    2 large tomatoes, washed, tops removed, and hulled
    1 small bread stick

For Dessert
    1 nectarine

Instructions: In a medium mixing bowl, combine tuna, mayonnaise, celery, and onion. Stuff into tomatoes and serve. Serve bread stick on the side. Serve nectarine for dessert.

Late Afternoon: Zone Snack (see page 88)

Dinner: Chicken Marinara with Three-Bean Salad*

Ingredients

1½ cups green beans, washed, ends removed, and
    cut in half

¼ cup canned chickpeas, drained

¼ cup canned kidney beans, drained

1⅓ teaspoons olive oil

2 tablespoons cider vinegar, or to taste

1 teaspoon dried chives

1 teaspoon dried parsley

½ teaspoon freshly ground pepper, or to taste

1½ teaspoons dried basil

3 ounces boneless, skinless chicken breast cutlets

2 tablespoons prepared tomato sauce

¼ teaspoon garlic powder, or to taste

1 ounce low-fat mozzarella cheese, shredded

-----

*If possible, make the three-bean salad ahead of time (up to 2 days) and store, tightly sealed, in refrigerator.

For Dessert
   1 peach

Instructions: Preheat oven to 450°. In a large pot fitted with a steaming basket, bring 1 inch water to boil. Add green beans to the basket and steam until crisp-tender, 10 minutes. Remove from basket, drain, and combine with chickpeas and kidney beans. In a small mixing bowl, combine olive oil, vinegar, chives, parsley, pepper, and 1 teaspoon of the basil; experiment with the oil-vinegar ratio to taste. Toss with beans, cover, and refrigerate for 30 minutes. Place chicken in a large piece of foil. Top chicken with tomato sauce and sprinkle with the remaining ½ teaspoon basil, garlic powder, and cheese. Fold foil loosely over chicken, leaving ample space for air. Carefully turn up and seal the ends and the middle so that juices won't leak out. Bake in the preheated oven for 20 minutes. Remove from oven and carefully open foil to prevent steam burns. Serve with bean salad. Serve peach for dessert.

Late Evening: Zone Snack (see page 88)

ZONE SNACK GUIDE

   The following is just a sampling of a variety of Zone snacks you can create or use the food group listing as a template for creating your very own "customized"

Zone snacks. Your afternoon and late-evening snacks are critically important for your success and like a Zone meal include a balance of protein, carbohydrate, and fat to keep you in the Zone. When time is critical and you're busy on the go, prepare your snacks ahead of time and take them with you when you're away from home.

Deviled Eggs with Hummus
2 hard boiled eggs
¼ cup hummus
Slice eggs, discard yolks and fill with
    1 tablespoon hummus
Paprika to taste

Low-fat Cottage Cheese & Fruit
¼ cup of low-fat cottage cheese
⅓ cup "lite" fruit cocktail
1 macadamia nut or 3 almonds

Tomato Salad & Low-fat Cheese
2 tomatoes, diced
1 clove of garlic, minced
⅓ teaspoon olive oil
1 teaspoon chopped fresh basil leaves
1 oz. part-skim or "soft" cheese
balsamic vinegar to taste

Waldorf Salad
1 cup celery, sliced
¼ apple, diced

½ teaspoon "lite" mayonnaise
1 pecan half, crushed
1 oz. part-skim or "soft" cheese on the side

Low-fat Yogurt & Nuts
½ cup plain low-fat yogurt
1 teaspoon slivered almonds or 1 macadamia nut

Chips & Salsa
½ oz. baked tortilla chips
1 tablespoon salsa
1 oz. low-fat cheese
1 tablespoon guacamole

Mini Pita Pizza
½ mini pita pocket topped with:
1 tablespoon tomato sauce
⅓ teaspoon olive oil
1 oz. part-skim mozzarella

Spinach Salad
1 hard boiled egg, sliced
1 large spinach salad:
5 cups raw spinach
⅓ chopped onion
1 cup chopped mushrooms
½ raw tomato
⅓ teaspoon olive oil
balsamic vinegar to taste

Crabmeat Salad Sandwiches

1½ oz. crabmeat

1 teaspoon "lite" mayonnaise

½ mini pita pocket cut in triangles

Veggies & Dip

Mix 2 oz. tofu with:

⅓ teaspoon olive oil and a sprinkle of dry onion
soup mix

1 cup sliced raw vegetables

Low-fat Cottage Cheese & Tomato

¼ cup low-fat cottage cheese

2 tomatoes, sliced

1 tablespoon guacamole

Chef Salad Snack

1 oz. sliced turkey or ham

1 tossed garden salad*

⅓ teaspoon olive oil and ⅔ teaspoon balsamic
vinegar dressing for the salad

Taco Salad

1 oz. ground turkey cooked with small amount of
cooking spray and a small amount of taco
seasoning

1 tablespoon salsa

1 tossed garden salad*

---

*See recipe for garden salad

1 tablespoon guacamole
Top salad with cooked ground turkey and avocado.

Ham & Fruit
4 slices 97% fat-free deli ham
½ apple
1 macadamia nut

Applesauce & Low-fat Cheese
⅓ cup applesauce
1 oz. low-fat cheese

Garden Salad
2 cups lettuce
⅓ bell pepper
1 tomato, sliced
The following ingredients are optional: ¼ cup
sliced cucumber; ¼ cup diced celery; ¼ cup
sliced mushrooms or 1 slice of onion.

Berries & Low-fat Cheese
½ cup blueberries or 1 cup strawberries
1 oz. low-fat or "soft" cheese

Cheese & Grapes
1 oz. part-skim mozzarella string cheese
½ cup grapes

Tuna Salad & Cracker
1 oz. tuna in spring water, drained
1 green olive, sliced

1 teaspoon lite mayonnaise
Mix above ingredients well
1 whole grain cracker
4 cucumber spears

Wine & Cheese
4 oz. red or white wine
1 oz. low-fat or "soft" cheese

Hot Dog
1 soy hot dog
1 6-inch tortilla
1 teaspoon mayonnaise or 1 tablespoon guacamole

Tuna Salad
1 oz. tuna in spring water, drained
1 garden salad*
⅔ teaspoon olive oil and 1 tablespoon
    vinegar dressing

You can create an infinite variety of your very own Zone-favorable snacks. Pick and choose one item from each food group below. It's as easy as 1–2–3.

Proteins
¼ cup of low-fat cottage cheese
1 oz. part-skim or "lite" mozzarella
2½ oz. part-skim or "lite" ricotta cheese
1 oz. sliced meats (turkey, ham, etc.)

---

*See recipe for garden salad

1 oz. tuna packed in water
1 oz. low-fat, part-skim, or "soft" cheese

Carbohydrates

½ apple
3 apricots
1 kiwi
1 tangerine
⅓ cup "lite" fruit cocktail
½ pear
1 cup strawberries
¾ cup blackberries
½ orange
½ cup grapes
8 cherries
½ nectarine
1 peach
1 plum
½ cup peaches
½ cup crushed pineapple
1 cup raspberries
½ cup blueberries
½ grapefruit

Fats

3 olives (green or black)
1 macadamia nut
1 tablespoon guacamole
3 almonds
6 peanuts
2 pecan halves

DINING OUT: YOUR ZONE AWAY FROM HOME

Now that you've got the tools for making Zone meals and using the Top Zone foods, you may want some general pointers to help you stick with the Zone Diet in everyday life. Can you still go to restaurants and follow the Zone Diet? The answer is a resounding yes!

Although I'm always drumming into your head that food is a drug, I also want food to be the ultimate pleasure. You should be salivating over your Zone meals and treating yourself to a nice dinner at your favorite restaurant. The sheer enjoyment of food is an integral part of the Zone plan, and I don't want to deny you any of the eating pleasures you've experienced in the past. All you need to do is follow some simple guidelines, and you can eat the way you'd like and stay in the Zone. You *can* have it both ways!

Most restaurants simply provide too much food, especially low-quality (i.e., high-glycemic load) carbohydrates like breads, pasta, and rice. It's cheaper for them to fill you up on starches, but it's hormonal disaster for you. Your goal is to transform your favorite restaurant meal into a Zone Meal. Follow these simple tips and it's automatic.

1. **Eat ahead of time.** Have a Zone snack less than two hours before you go to the restaurant. It's much easier to dine in the Zone and make the right food choices if your blood sugar is stable.

2. **Skip the bread.** When you are seated, simply ask your server not to bring any bread or rolls to the table. If you need something before your main course, have a glass of wine and a protein appetizer (like smoked salmon or shrimp cocktail). Sipping your wine, determine the protein entrée you plan to eat (such as grilled chicken or fish).

3. **Substitute for low-quality side dishes.** Ask your waiter if you can replace any side dishes that are low-quality carbohydrates (pasta, rice, grains, or other starches) with high-quality carbohydrates like steamed vegetables.

4. **Create a Zone-size meal.** When the meal arrives, cut a serving out of your protein entrée that's as big as the size and thickness of your palm. Ask your waiter to wrap the rest of your entrée up so you can take it home. Of course you still eat all of the high-quality carbohydrates that came with the entrée.

5. **Divvy up dessert.** If you want a rich dessert, eat only half and give the other half to your dining partner. Of course, if you opt for fresh fruit, you can eat the whole thing.

6. **Give yourself a little leeway.** Finally, if you consume too many carbohydrates or too many calories at a meal, don't worry that you've done irreparable damage. You can reset your hormonal system if you make sure your next meal is a Zone meal.

You can use these tips at any restaurant, but here are some additional hints for dining out in popular specialty restaurants.

Chinese

Forget the rice, and you have all the makings of a great Zone meal. Grilled fish or chicken, stir-fried chicken, or tofu dishes are great sources of protein. Choose a protein dish that's piled high with abundant levels of high-quality carbohydrates, such as vegetables, to accompany your high-quality Zone protein choice.

Italian

This is always a potential Zone disaster because of the heaping amounts of pasta and bread piled on your plate. Try the chicken or fish entrees served with extra vegetables instead of pasta. Drizzle on some olive oil to enhance the flavor of your salads and cooked vegetables. If you want pasta, have it as a very small side dish. I wouldn't recommend the side dish of pasta, though, if you're planning on drinking wine, since you'll eat far too many carbohydrates to have a Zone meal.

Japanese

Japanese cuisine is more Zone balanced than what you typically find in a Chinese restaurant, but you still should avoid the rice. Fish and tofu entrees with abundant amounts of steamed vegetables are great. Even sushi is not a bad balance of protein and carbohydrate. (Helpful hint: A breaded protein dish like tempura is not a high-quality Zone protein choice.)

Mexican

This is another potential Zone disaster area because of the large amounts of low-quality carbohydrates, especially the chips, refried beans, rice, and tortillas. You can stay in the Zone, though, if you choose the chicken fajitas. Always ask for corn instead of flour tortillas to decrease your carbohydrate intake, and for extra vegetables in place of the rice or refried beans. Don't forget to dab on a little guacamole, which is a great source of monounsaturated fat.

French

If you're eating in a gourmet French restaurant, you'll probably be in Zone heaven. You'll be served a small serving of protein piled with plenty of crisp colorful vegetables lightly dressed in olive oil. Enjoy the wine and the meal.

Pizza Parlors

Yes, you *can* still eat pizza in the Zone. It's not the highest-quality meal you can find, but it's OK on occasion. Order the thin crust pizza instead of the thick crust and make sure you have a protein-rich topping like cheese, chicken or even anchovies. Then eat the topping of every slice, but only eat every other crust. To make your pizza more satisfying, order extra vegetables as a topping.

Dining Out for Business Travelers

Eating on the road is one of the most stressful events for any business traveler, especially in new locales. At every meal use the basic guidelines outlined above. Here's a sample of some high-quality Zone meals that are always available regardless of where you're staying.

Breakfast
Egg-white omelet with a side order of oatmeal. This is the ultimate power breakfast. Just don't eat the toast and the hash brown potatoes.

Lunch
Chicken Caesar salad with fresh fruit for dessert.

Dinner
Grilled fish with extra vegetables in place of the starch. Have fresh fruit for dessert. Consider having

---

a glass of wine with the dinner, and always pass on the rolls.

Road Snacks

Have 1 ounce of sliced turkey or of low-fat cheese with half a piece of fruit.

PART IV

Zone Food Blocks for Prepared Meals

If time is of the essence, then prepared (either frozen or in cans) meals can be a godsend. However, be aware that many of these prepared meals can take you quickly out of the Zone if they aren't balanced with regard to Zone Food Blocks.

I have already provided a few examples in Part II, but this section goes into even greater detail.

As I said earlier, the food industry is doing everything in its considerable power to entice you to buy prepackaged foods. As a result, it's a war out there, and the only advantage you have is to have knowledge. In this section, I have taken a good number of prepared meals and broken them down into their individual Zone Food Blocks. What you are going to find is that most of your favorite packaged foods are extremely rich in carbohydrates and fat (and that means a lot of trans fat to get a longer shelf life for the products).

Another problem with packaged foods is that the

primary sources of carbohydrates are high-glycemic load carbohydrates (grains and starches). Not only are they much cheaper than low glycemic load carbohydrates (vegetables and fruits), but they can be made into virtually anything that will last forever. That's great for the food companies, but a terrible disaster for your hormones.

Here is a quick way to turn the tables on the food giants. Simply add enough Zone protein blocks to balance out the carbohydrates so that you will lessen the insulin impact these packaged foods normally have on your body. Of course you still have to contend with the extra fat (including the trans fats) in packaged foods, but that is the price you pay for convenience.

FROZEN MEALS

The following frozen meals can fit into the Zone, but sometimes need a little tinkering. Therefore, read the food labels carefully, because they are constantly changing.

Stouffer's Lean Cuisine

Beef Peppercorn
Grilled Chicken
Chicken and Vegetables

Healthy Choice

Grilled Chicken Sonoma (sprinkle a little Parmesan cheese on top)

Grilled Peppercorn Beef Patty

Garlic Chicken Milano (sprinkle a little Parmesan cheese on top)

Turkey Breast Medallions (add 2 teaspoons slivered almonds and have ¼ cup grapes for dessert)

Marie Callender

Grilled Turkey Breast Strips

Swedish Meatballs (a little high in fat)

Weight Watchers (these meals need quite a bit of work to get them into the Zone)

Fiesta Chicken (add 2 teaspoons slivered almonds and either 1 ounce low-fat cheese or 1 additional ounce of chicken)

Creamy Rigatoni with Broccoli Chicken (add 2 ounces chicken and 9 sliced olives)

Now that you have the idea, here are hundreds of prepared meals with the number of Zone Blocks in each. By adding enough of the right Blocks, you can make any prepared meal into a balanced Zone meal.

PREPARED MEAL ITEM	SPECIFICATIONS	BRAND NAME	SERVING SIZE	PROTEIN BLOCKS	CARBOHYDRATE BLOCKS	FAT BLOCKS
Alfredo Sauce		Ragu	1/4 cup	0	0	3
		Progresso	1/4 cup	1	0	5
	three cheese	Lawry's	3 Tbs.	0	0	1
	refrigerated	Contadina	1/4 cup	1	0	6
	refrigerated	Contadina Light	1/4 cup	1	1	2
Alfredo Sauce mix		Knorr	1/3 pkg.	0	1	1
		Spice Island	1/2 pkg.	0	0	1
Amaranth entree	canned	Health Valley Fast Menu	1 cup	1	3	0
Angel Hair pasta entree	frozen	Lean Cuisine	1 pkg.	1	3	1
	frozen	Smart Ones	1 pkg.	1	3	1
	frozen w/sausage	Marie Callender's	1 pkg.	2	4	5
Angel Hair pasta mix	chicken	Golden Saute	1/2 pkg. dry	1	5	1
	w/herbs	Noodle Roni	1 cup prepared	1	4	4
	parmesan	Golden Saute	1/2 cup, dry	1	4	2
		Noodle Roni Parmesano	1 cup prepared	1	4	5
Apple Fritters	frozen	Mrs. Paul's	2 pcs.	1	4	4

Apple Pastry	frozen, dumpling	Pepperidge Farm	1 pc.	0	5	4
	pocket	Tastykake	1 pc.	0	4	8
	puffs	Entenmann's	1 pc.	0	4	4
	frozen, squares	Pepperidge Farm	1 pc.	0	3	3
Bean Dishes, mix	Italian	Knorr Cup	1 pkg.	1	5	1
Bean Entree, frozen	white Parisian	Weight Watchers	10 oz.	2	1	3
Bean Loaf	frozen	Natural Touch	1 slice	1	1	3
Bean Salad	deli style	S&W	1/2 cup	1	2	0
	marinated	S&W	1/2 cup	0	1	0
	three bean	Green Giant	1/2 cup	0	1	0
	three bean	Hanover	1/3 cup	0	2	0
Beans and Franks		Campbell's	1 cup	3	3	4
		Hormel	7 1/2 oz.	2	3	4
		Kid's Kitchen	7 1/2 oz.	2	3	4
		Libby's Diner	7 3/4 oz.	2	3	5
		Van de Kamp's Beanie Weenee	1 cup	2	3	5
	baked	Van de Kamp's Beanie Weenee	1 cup	3	5	5

PREPARED MEAL ITEM	SPECIFICATIONS	BRAND NAME	SERVING SIZE	PROTEIN BLOCKS	CARBOHYDRATE BLOCKS	FAT BLOCKS
Beans and Franks (cont'd)	barbeque	Van de Kamp's Beanie Weenee	1 cup	2	4	3
	chili	Van de Kamp's Beanie Weenee	1 can	2	2	4
Beef Dinner, frozen	and broccoli	Swanson	1 pkg	2	5	3
	and broccoli	Swanson Hungry Man	1 pkg	4	7	5
	chicken fried steak	Banquet	1 pkg	4	7	15
	chicken fried steak	Marie Callender's	1 pkg	3	7	10
	chicken fried steak w/gravy	Swanson	1 pkg	5	5	8
	and gravy	Swanson	1 pkg	2	4	2
	and peppers Cantonese	Healthy Choice	1 pkg	2	1	2
	pot roast, Yankee	The Budget Gourmet Light & Healthy	1 pkg	3	3	2
	pot roast, Yankee	Healthy Choice	1 pkg	3	4	2
	pot roast, Yankee	Swanson	1 pkg	1	3	2
	pot roast, Yankee	Swanson Hungry Man	1 pkg	2	4	4
	roast beef sandwich, smothered	Swanson	1 pkg	2	5	4

Salisbury steak	Banquet	1 pkg	4	5	15
Salisbury steak	The Budget Gourmet	1 pkg	3	3	3
	Light & Healthy				
Salisbury steak	Healthy Choice	1 pkg	3	5	2
Salisbury steak	Swanson	1 pkg	4	4	7
Salisbury steak	Swanson Hungry Man	1 pkg	7	4	11
Salisbury steak, con queso	Patio	1 pkg	3	3	7
sirloin	The Budget Gourmet	1 pkg	3	4	2
	Light & Healthy				
	Special Recipe				
sirloin, chopped w/gravy	Swanson	1 pkg	2	3	3
sirloin, meatballs and gravy	The Budget Gourmet	1 pkg	3	4	3
	Light & Healthy				
sirloin, tips	Swanson Hungry Man	1 pkg	4	4	5
sirloin, tips, w/noodles	Swanson	1 pkg	2	3	3
sirloin, in wine sauce	The Budget Gourmet	1 pkg	3	3	2
	Light & Healthy				

PREPARED MEAL ITEM	SPECIFICATIONS	BRAND NAME	SERVING SIZE	PROTEIN BLOCKS	CARBOHYDRATE BLOCKS	FAT BLOCKS
Beef Dinner, frozen (cont'd)	Stroganoff	Healthy Choice	1 pkg	3	5	2
	teriyaki	The Budget Gourmet Light & Healthy	1 pkg	3	4	2
	tips	Healthy Choice	1 pkg	3	3	2
	tips, sauce	Healthy Choice	1 pkg	3	4	2
Beef Entree, canned	chow mein	La Choy Bi-Pack	1 cup	1	1	1
	goulash	Hormel	7 1/2 oz. can	2	2	4
	pepper steak, Oriental	La Choy Bi-Pack	1 cup	2	1	1
	pepper steak, Oriental, w/noodles	La Choy Bi-Pack	1 cup	3	2	1
	pot roast	Dinty Moore American Classics	10 oz.	4	2	1
	roast, w/mashed potato	Dinty Moore American Classics	10 oz.	3	3	2
	Salisbury steak	Dinty Moore American Classics	10 oz.	3	2	5
	stew	Dinty Moore	1 cup	2	2	5
	stew	Dinty Moore, Can	7 1/2 oz.	2	1	3
	stew	Dinty Moore, Cup	7 1/2 oz.	2	1	3

	stew	Dinty Moore American Classics	10 oz.	2	2	4
	stew	Hormel Micro cup	7 1/2 oz.	2	1	3
	stew	Hunt's Homestyle	1 cup	2	2	2
	stew	Libby's Diner	7 3/4 oz.	2	2	7
	stew	Nalley's	7 1/2 oz.	1	2	3
	stew	Nalley's Big Chunk	1 cup	2	2	4
	stew, burger	Dinty Moore Hearty Cup	7 1/2 oz.	2	2	4
	w/peppers, onions, rice	Mountain House	1 cup	2	3	2
Beef Entree, freeze dried	stew	Mountain House	1 cup	1	2	1
	Stroganoff, w/noodles	Mountain House	1 cup	1	3	3
	teriyaki, w/rice	Mountain House	1 cup	2	4	1
Beef Entree, frozen	barbeque, mesquite	Healthy Choice	1 pkg.	3	4	1
	broccoli, Beijing	Healthy Choice	1 pkg.	3	6	1
	Cantonese	The Budget Gourmet	1 pkg.	2	4	3
	chipped	Banquet Topper	4 oz.	1	1	1

PREPARED MEAL ITEM	SPECIFICATIONS	BRAND NAME	SERVING SIZE	PROTEIN BLOCKS	CARBOHYDRATE BLOCKS	FAT BLOCKS
Beef Entree, frozen (cont'd)	chipped, creamed	Stouffer's	4 1/2 oz.	1	1	4
	ground, w/rice	Goya	1 pkg.	4	12	12
	mesquite, w/rice	Lean Cuisine Café Classics	1 pkg.	2	4	2
	Oriental	The Budget Gourmet, Light & Healthy	1 pkg.	2	4	3
	Oriental	Lean Cuisine Café Classics	1 pkg.	2	3	3
	Oriental	Stouffer's Lunch Express	1 pkg.	2	4	3
	patty	Swanson Fun Feast	1 pkg.	4	5	6
	patty, charbroiled, gravy and	Morton	1 pkg.	2	2	5
	patty, gravy and	Banquet	1 pkg.	2	2	7
	patty, mushroom, gravy and	Banquet	1 patty	1	1	4
	patty, onion gravy and	Banquet	1 patty	1	1	5
	pepper steak	The Budget Gourmet	1 pkg.	3	4	3
	pepper steak	Stouffer's	1 pkg.	2	5	3
	pepper steak	Weight Watchers	1 pkg.	3	3	2

pepper steak, Oriental	Healthy Choice	1 pkg.	3	3	1
pie or pot pie	Banquet	1 pkg.	1	4	5
pie or pot pie	Stouffer's	1 pkg.	3	4	9
pie or pot pie	Swanson	1 pkg.	5	4	8
pie or pot pie	Swanson Hungry Man	1 pkg.	8	7	13
pot pie, Yankee	Marie Callender's	1 pkg.	2	6	15
pot roast, w/potatoes	Lean Cuisine	1 pkg.	2	2	2
pot roast, w/potatoes	Stouffer's Homestyle	1 pkg.	3	2	3
roast	Healthy Choice Hearty Handfuls	6 oz.	2	5	2
roast, open face	The Budget Gourmet	1 pkg.	2	3	6
Salisbury steak	Banquet	1 pkg.	2	3	5
Salisbury steak	Healthy Choice	1 pkg.	3	3	2
Salisbury steak	Lean Cuisine	1 pkg.	3	3	3
Salisbury steak	Stouffer's Homestyle	1 pkg.	3	3	6
Salisbury steak, gravy and	Banquet	1 patty	2	1	5
Salisbury steak, gravy and	Banquet Toppers	5 oz	1	1	5
Salisbury steak, gravy and	Morton	1 pkg.	1	2	3

PREPARED MEAL ITEM	SPECIFICATIONS	BRAND NAME	SERVING SIZE	PROTEIN BLOCKS	CARBOHYDRATE BLOCKS	FAT BLOCKS
Beef Entrée, frozen *(cont'd)*	Salisbury steak, gravy, mashed potato	Swanson	1 pkg.	4	2	6
	Salisbury steak, grilled	Weight Watchers	1 pkg.	3	2	3
	Salisbury steak, sirloin	The Budget Gourmet Light & Healthy	1 pkg.	3	3	2
	shredded, w/rice	Goya	1 pkg.	5	13	8
	sirloin, cheddar melt	The Budget Gourmet	1 pkg.	2	3	7
	sirloin in herb sauce	The Budget Gourmet Light & Healthy	1 pkg.	3	3	2
	sirloin, peppercorn	Lean Cuisine Café Classics	1 pkg.	2	2	2
	sirloin, roast supreme	The Budget Gourmet	1 pkg.	2	3	4
	sirloin tips, and noodles	Swanson	1 pkg.	2	2	3
	sirloin tips, w/vegetables	The Budget Gourmet	1 pkg.	2	2	4
	sliced	Banquet Country	1 pkg.	4	2	2
	sliced, gravy and	Banquet	2 slices	2	1	1

sliced, gravy and	Banquet Topper	4 oz.	1	0	1
steak, chicken fried	Banquet, Country	1 pkg.	2	4	7
Philly	Healthy Choice	6 oz.	2	5	2
	Hearty Handfuls				
stew	Banquet	1 cup	2	1	1
stew w/rice	Goya	1 pkg.	5	13	6
stir-fry	Tyson Kit	1 cup	2	3	1
Stroganoff	The Budget Gourmet	1 pkg.	3	3	2
	Light & Healthy				
Stroganoff	Stouffer's	1 pkg.	3	3	7
tips, Francois	Healthy Choice	1 pkg.	3	4	2
Beef Hash, canned	Broadcast Morning Classics	1 cup	1	2	4
	Original				
corned beef	Castleberry's	1 cup	3	2	9
	Dinty Moore Cup	7 1/2 oz.	3	2	7
	Goya	1 cup	2	2	10
	Libby's	1 cup	3	2	12

PREPARED MEAL ITEM	SPECIFICATIONS	BRAND NAME	SERVING SIZE	PROTEIN BLOCKS	CARBOHYDRATE BLOCKS	FAT BLOCKS
Beef Hash, canned		Mary Kitchen	1 cup	3	2	8
(cont'd)		Nalley's	1 cup	3	2	11
	roast beef	Libby's	1 cup	3	2	11
		Mary Kitchen	1 cup	3	2	8
	sausage flavor	Broadcast Morning Classics	1 cup	1	2	4
Beef Sandwich, frozen	barbeque	Hormel Quick Meal	1 pc.	2	6	2
	barbeque	Hot Pockets	1 pc.	2	6	1
	broccoli	Lean Pockets	1 pc.	1	5	1
	cheddar	Hot Pockets	1 pc.	2	5	2
	cheeseburger	Hormel Quick Meal	1 pc.	3	5	2
	cheeseburger, bacon	Hormel Quick Meal	1 pc.	3	4	7
	cheeseburger, chili	Hormel Quick Meal	1 pc.	3	4	8
	fajita	Hot Pockets	1 pc.	2	4	6
	hamburger	Hormel Quick Meal	1 pc.	3	4	5
	steak, biscuit	Hormel Quick Meal	1 pc.	2	4	5

Bowtie entree, frozen	steak, mushroom	Mrs. Paterson's Aussie Pie	1 pc.	2	4	8
	and chicken	Lean Cuisine Café Classics	1 pkg.	3	3	2
	mushroom Marsala	Weight Watchers	1 pkg.	2	3	3
Broccoli pocket	and cheddar, frozen	Ken & Robert's Veggie Pockets	1 pc.	1	4	3
Broccoli pot pie	w/cheddar, frozen	Amy's	7 1/2 oz.	2	5	7
Broccoli-cheese in pastry		Pepperidge Farm	1 pc.	1	2	5
Burrito, frozen	bean, black	Amy's	1 pc. or pkg.	1	6	3
	bean and cheese	Old El Paso	1 pc. or pkg.	2	5	3
	bean and cheese	Tina's	1 pc. or pkg.	2	5	3
	bean and rice	Amy's	1 pc. or pkg.	1	4	2
	bean, rice, and cheese	Amy's	1 pc. or pkg.	1	4	3
	beef	Hormel Quick meal	1 pc. or pkg.	1	4	4
	beef	Tina's Red Hot	1 pc. or pkg.	2	5	5
	beef, nacho	Patio Britos	6 oz.	2	5	6
	beef and bean	Patio Britos	6 oz.	2	5	6
	beef and bean, hot	Old El Paso	1 pc. or pkg.	2	5	3

PREPARED MEAL ITEM	SPECIFICATIONS	BRAND NAME	SERVING SIZE	PROTEIN BLOCKS	CARBOHYDRATE BLOCKS	FAT BLOCKS
Burrito, frozen *(cont'd)*	beef and bean, medium	Old El Paso	1 pc. or pkg.	2	5	3
	beef and bean, mild	Old El Paso	1 pc. or pkg.	2	5	3
	beef and bean, steak	Don Miguel	1 pc. or pkg.	2	6	3
	cheese	Hormel Quick Meal	1 pc. or pkg.	1	4	2
	cheese, nacho	Patio Britos	1 pc. or pkg.	1	5	4
	chicken	Don Miguel	1 pc. or pkg.	2	5	3
	chicken, and cheese, spicy	Patio Britos	1 pc. or pkg.	2	5	5
	chicken son queso	Healthy Choice	1 pc. or pkg.	2	4	2
	chili, red	Hormel Quick Meal	1 pc. or pkg.	1	4	4
	pizza, cheese	Old El Paso	1 pc. or pkg.	2	3	3
	pizza, pepperoni	Old El Paso	1 pc. or pkg.	2	3	3
	pizza, sausage	Old El Paso	1 pc. or pkg.	2	4	3
	black bean	Amy's	1 pkg.	1	4	2
Burrito, breakfast, frozen	egg, scrambled	Swanson Great Starts Original	1 pkg.	2	3	3

Food	Description	Brand	Serving	P	C	F
	egg, scrambled, w/bacon	Swanson Great Starts	1 pkg.	2	3	4
	ham and cheese	Swanson Great Starts	1 pkg.	1	3	2
	hot and spicy	Swanson Great Starts	1 pkg.	2	3	2
	pizza, w/cheese, pepperoni	Swanson Great Starts	1 pkg.	2	3	3
	sausage	Swanson Great Starts	1 pkg.	3	3	4
Burrito dinner, frozen	beef	Chi-Chi's Burro	15 oz.	4	7	6
	chicken	Chi-Chi's Burro	15 oz.	4	7	5
Cabbage, stuffed	frozen, w/potato	Lean Cuisine	9 1/2 oz.	2	2	2
Calzone refrigerated	cheese	Stefano's	6-oz. pc.	3	4	9
	pepperoni	Stefano's	6-oz. pc.	3	5	9
	spinach	Stefano's	6-oz. pc.	3	5	6
Cannelloni dinner	frozen, w/potato	Amy's	10 oz.	2	3	4
Cannelloni entree	frozen, cheese	Lean Cuisine	9 oz.	3	3	2
Cheese Sandwich	frozen, grilled	Swanson Fun Feast	1 pkg.	4	6	7
Chicken dinner, frozen	barbeque, mesquite	The Budget Gourmet	1 pkg.	3	3	2
	barbeque, mesquite	Healthy Choice Light and Healthy	1 pkg.	3	5	1

PREPARED MEAL ITEM	SPECIFICATIONS	BRAND NAME	SERVING SIZE	PROTEIN BLOCKS	CARBOHYDRATE BLOCKS	FAT BLOCKS
Chicken dinner,	boneless	Swanson Hungry Man	1 pkg.	6	8	9
frozen (cont'd)	breaded, country	Healthy Choice	1 pkg.	3	0	2
	broccoli Alfredo	Healthy Choice	1 pkg.	3	5	3
	Cantonese	Healthy Choice	1 pkg.	3	3	0
	Dijon	Healthy Choice	1 pkg.	3	4	1
	fried	Banquet Extra Helping	1 pkg.	5	7	13
	fried, country, w/gravy	Marie Callender's	1 pkg.	4	7	9
	fried, dark	Swanson	1 pkg.	6	5	9
	fried, dark	Swanson Budget	1 pkg.	5	5	7
	fried, dark	Swanson Hungry Man	1 pkg.	9	7	14
	fried, Southern	Banquet Extra Helping	1 pkg.	5	6	12
	fried, white	Banquet Extra Helping	1 pkg.	6	7	14
	fried, white	Swanson	1 pkg.	6	5	9
	fried, white, mostly	Swanson Hungry Man	1 pkg.	9	8	13
	glazed, Southwestern	Healthy Choice	1 pkg.	3	5	1

grilled, patties	Swanson Hungry Man	1 pkg.	4	6	2
grilled, white in garlic sauce	Swanson	1 pkg.	1	3	2
herb, country	Healthy Choice	1 pkg.	3	4	1
herbed	The Budget Gourmet Light & Healthy	1 pkg.	4	3	3
honey mustard	The Budget Gourmet Light & Healthy	1 pkg.	3	4	2
nuggets	Swanson	1 pkg.	4	5	6
parmigiana	Banquet Extra Helping	1 pkg.	3	6	11
parmigiana	The Budget Gourmet Light & Healthy	1 pkg.	3	3	3
parmigiana	Healthy Choice	1 pkg.	3	5	1
parmigiana	Marie Callender's	1 pkg.	4	6	9
parmigiana	Swanson	1 pkg.	4	4	6
parmigiana	Swanson Budget	1 pkg.	4	3	6
pasta and	Swanson Budget	1 pkg.	2	3	4

PREPARED MEAL ITEM	SPECIFICATIONS	BRAND NAME	SERVING SIZE	PROTEIN BLOCKS	CARBOHYDRATE BLOCKS	FAT BLOCKS
Chicken dinner, frozen *(cont'd)*	picante	Healthy Choice	1 pkg.	3	3	1
	roasted, herb	The Budget Gourmet Light & Healthy	1 pkg.	2	3	2
	roasted, herb	Swanson	1 pkg.	1	4	2
	roasted, herb, mashed potatoes	Marie Callender's	1 pkg.	6	3	14
	sweet and sour	Healthy Choice	1 pkg.	3	4	2
	tenders platter	Swanson	1 pkg.	3	4	4
	teriyaki	The Budget Gourmet Light & Healthy	1 pkg.	3	4	2
	teriyaki	Healthy Choice	1 pkg.	3	4	1
Chicken entree, canned	a la king	Swanson Main Dish	1 cup	5	2	7
	a la king	Top Shelf	10 oz.	3	5	4
	breast glazed	Top Shelf	10 oz.	3	2	2
	and broccoli	Healthy Choice Hearty Handfuls	6 oz.	2	5	2

cacciatore	Top Shelf	10 oz.	3	3	1
chow mein	La Choy Bi-Pack	1 cup	1	1	1
chow mein	La Choy Entree	1 cup	1	0	1
and dumplings	Dinty Moore Cup	7 1/2 oz.	2	2	2
and dumplings	Swanson Main Dish	1 cup	3	2	4
fiesta	Top Shelf	10 oz.	4	5	5
w/mashed potatoes	Dinty Moore American Classics	10 oz.	3	3	1
and noodles	Dinty Moore American Classics	10 oz.	3	3	3
Oriental, w/noodles	La Choy	1 cup	2	1	2
and pasta	Chef Boyardee Bowl	7 1/2 oz.	2	2	0
spicy	La Choy Szechwan Bi-Pack	1 cup	1	1	1
stew	Dinty Moore	1 cup	2	2	4
stew	Dinty Moore Cup	7 1/2 oz.	1	2	3
stew	Swanson Main Dish	1 cup	3	2	3
sweet and sour	La Choy Bi-Pack	1 cup	1	3	1
teriyaki	La Choy Bi-Pack	1 cup	1	1	1
Chicken entree, freeze-dried					
a la king and noodles	Mountain House	1 cup	3	3	3

PREPARED MEAL ITEM	SPECIFICATIONS	BRAND NAME	SERVING SIZE	PROTEIN BLOCKS	CARBOHYDRATE BLOCKS	FAT BLOCKS
Chicken entree, freeze-dried (cont'd)	honey lime, w/rice	Mountain House	1 cup	1	5	1
	noodles and	Mountain House	1 cup	2	3	1
	Polynesian w/rice	Mountain House	1 cup	1	4	1
	rice and	Mountain House	1 cup	1	5	3
	stew	Mountain House	1 cup	2	2	3
	teriyaki, w/rice	Mountain House	1 cup	1	4	1
Chicken entree, frozen, see also Chicken entree, refrigerated	a la king	Banquet Toppers	4 1/2 oz. bag	1	1	1
	a la king	Stouffer's	1 pkg.	2	4	3
	Alfredo	Stouffer's Lunch Express	1 pkg.	3	3	6
	au gratin	The Budget Gourmet Light & Healthy	1 pkg.	3	3	3
	baked and gravy, whipped potato	Stouffer's Homestyle	1 pkg.	3	2	4

baked, whipped potato	Lean Cuisine	1 pkg.	3	3	2
barbeque, glazed	Weight Watchers	1 pkg.	3	3	1
barbeque, honey, w/potato, vegetables	Tyson	1 pkg.	3	5	5
barbeque style	Banquet	1 pkg.	3	4	4
barbeque w/potato, vegetables	Tyson BBQ	1 pkg.	3	5	3
biryani	Curry Classics	1 pkg.	4	6	4
blackened	Tyson	1 pkg.	2	4	1
breaded cutlet, pasta marinara	Celentano	1 pkg.	3	3	6
breast breaded	Tyson	2 pcs.	2	2	3
breast breaded, southern	Tyson Breast Fillets	2 pcs.	2	1	2
breast, in wine sauce	Lean Cuisine Café Classics	1 pkg.	2	2	2
breast tenders	Banquet	3 pcs.	2	2	5
breast tenders	Tyson	5 pcs.	2	1	5
breast tenders, Southern	Banquet	3 pcs.	2	2	5

PREPARED MEAL ITEM	SPECIFICATIONS	BRAND NAME	SERVING SIZE	PROTEIN BLOCKS	CARBOHYDRATE BLOCKS	FAT BLOCKS
Chicken entree, frozen, see also Chicken entree, refrigerated (cont'd)	w/broccoli and cheese	Tyson	1 pkg.	3	2	4
	cacciatore	Healthy Choice	1 pkg.	3	3	1
	Calypso	Lean Cuisine Café Classics	1 pkg.	2	4	2
	carbonara	Lean Cuisine Café Classics	1 pkg.	3	3	3
	chow mein	Banquet	1 pkg.	1	3	2
	chow mein	Chun King	1 pkg.	2	5	5
	chow mein	Lean Cuisine	1 pkg.	2	3	2
	chow mein	Smart Ones	1 pkg.	2	3	1
	chow mein	Stouffer's Lunch Express	1 pkg.	2	4	1
	chunks, breaded	Country Skillet	5 pcs.	2	2	6
	chunks, breaded	Tyson Breast Chunks	6 pcs.	2	1	5
	chunks, breaded	Tyson Chick'n Chunks	6 pcs.	2	1	7
	chunks, breaded, and cheddar	Banquet	4 pcs.	2	1	6
	chunks, breaded, Southern	Banquet	5 pcs.	2	2	6

chunks, breaded, Southern	Country Skillet	5 pcs.	2	2	5
chunks, breaded, Southern	Tyson Chick'n Chunks	6 pcs.	1	1	6
Cordon Bleu	Weight Watchers	1 pkg.	2	3	2
creamed	Stouffer's	1 pkg.	2	1	7
creamy and broccoli	Stouffer's	1 pkg.	3	3	5
crouquettes	Goya	3 pcs.	2	3	4
drumlets	Swanson Fun Feast	1 pkg.	5	5	8
and dumplings	Banquet Family Size	1 cup	2	2	5
and dumplings	Banquet Home Style	1 pkg.	2	4	3
enchilada, see "Enchilada Entree"			0	0	0
escalloped, and noodles	Stouffer's	1 pkg.	2	3	9
fajita, see "Fajita entree"			0	0	0
fettuccine	The Budget Gourmet	1 pkg.	3	3	6
fettuccine	Lean Cuisine	1 pkg.	3	3	2
fettuccine	Stouffer's Homestyle	1 pkg.	4	3	5
fettuccine	Weight Watchers	1 pkg.	3	4	2

PREPARED MEAL ITEM	SPECIFICATIONS	BRAND NAME	SERVING SIZE	PROTEIN BLOCKS	CARBOHYDRATE BLOCKS	FAT BLOCKS
Chicken entree, frozen, see also Chicken entree, refrigerated (cont'd)	fettuccine	Healthy Choice	1 pkg.	3	4	2
	w/broccoli and cheese	Lean Cuisine Lunch Express	1 pkg.	2	4	3
	fiesta	Lean Cuisine	1 pkg.	3	4	2
	fiesta	Smart Ones	1 pkg.	2	4	1
	Francais	Tyson	1 pkg.	3	2	3
	Francesca	Healthy Choice	1 pkg.	4	5	2
	French recipe	The Budget Gourmet Light & Healthy	1 pkg.	2	2	3
	fricassee, w/rice	Goya	1 pkg.	6	13	7
	fried	Banquet Meal	1 pkg.	3	3	9
	fried	Kid Cuisine High Flying	1 pkg.	3	5	6
	fried	Morton	1 pkg.	3	3	8
	fried	Swanson Fun Feast Frasslin'	1 pkg.	7	5	10
	fried, Southern	Banquet Meal	1 pkg.	3	4	10
	fried, whipped potato	Stouffer's Homestyle	1 pkg.	3	3	5
	fried, whipped potato	Swanson	1 pkg.	5	4	7

fried, white meat	Banquet Meal	1 pkg.	3	3	9
fried, pieces	Banquet Original	3 oz.	2	1	6
fried, pieces	Country Skillet	3 oz.	2	1	6
fried, breast	Banquet Original	5 1/2-oz. pc.	3	2	9
fried, country	Banquet	3 oz.	2	1	6
fried, drums and thighs	Banquet	3 oz.	2	1	6
fried, honey BBQ, skinless	Banquet	3 oz.	4	1	4
fried, hot 'n spicy	Banquet	3 oz.	2	1	6
fried, skinless	Banquet	3 oz.	3	1	4
fried, Southern	Banquet	3 oz.	2	1	6
fried, wing, hot and spicy	Banquet	4 oz.	2	0	5
fried rice	Tyson Kit	1 cup	2	4	1
garlic	Healthy Choice Hearty Handfuls	6 oz.	3	5	2
garlic, milano	Healthy Choice	1 pkg.	3	3	1
ginger, Hunan	Healthy Choice	1 pkg.	3	6	1
glazed, country	Healthy Choice	1 pkg.	2	3	1
glazed, w/rice,	Tyson	1 pkg.	2	3	2
broccoli, carrots					

PREPARED MEAL ITEM	SPECIFICATIONS	BRAND NAME	SERVING SIZE	PROTEIN BLOCKS	CARBOHYDRATE BLOCKS	FAT BLOCKS
Chicken entree, frozen, see also Chicken	glazed, w/vegetable rice	Lean Cuisine	1 pkg.	3	2	2
	grilled, angel hair pasta	Stouffer's Lunch Express	1 pkg.	3	4	4
entree, refrigerated	grilled, w/corn, beans	Tyson	1 pkg.	3	2	1
(cont'd)	grilled, Italian, w/linguine	Tyson	1 pkg.	3	2	1
	grilled, salsa	Lean Cuisine Café Classics	1 pkg.	2	3	2
	grilled, gumbo	Goya Asopao de Pollo	1 pkg.	2	2	1
	herb, w/radiatore, vegetables	Tyson	1 pkg.	3	5	2
	honey mustard	Lean Cuisine Café Classics	1 pkg.	2	4	2
	honey mustard	Healthy Choice	1 pkg.	3	4	1
	honey mustard	Smart Ones	1 pkg.	2	3	1
	honey mustard, w/gemelli	Tyson	1 pkg.	3	5	2
	imperial	Healthy Choice	1 pkg.	2	3	1
	Italian, w/fettuccine	Lean Cuisine	1 pkg.	3	3	2
	Kiev	Tyson	1 pkg.	3	4	8
	w/linguine	Stouffer's Lunch Express	1 pkg.	2	3	4

lo mein	Banquet		2	4	2
mandarin	The Budget Gourmet Light & Healthy	1 pkg.	2	4	2
mandarin	Lean Cuisine Lunch Express	1 pkg.	2	4	2
mandarin	Healthy Choice	1 pkg.	3	4	1
marinara, w/pasta	Tyson	1 pkg.	4	6	3
Marsala	The Budget Gourmet	1 pkg.	3	3	2
Marsala	Smart Ones	1 pkg.	1	2	1
Marsala, w/potato, carrots	Tyson	1 pkg.	2	2	2
Marsala and vegetables	Healthy Choice	1 pkg.	3	3	0
Mediterranean	Lean Cuisine Café Classics	1 pkg.	3	3	1
mesquite	Tyson	1 pkg.	3	4	2
Mexican, and rice	Stouffer's Lunch Express	1 pkg.	2	4	3
Mirabella	Smart Ones	1 pkg.	2	2	1
Monterey	Stouffer's Homestyle	1 pkg.	3	3	7
and mushroom	Healthy Choice Hearty Handfuls	6.1 oz.	2	5	1
w/mushroom sauce	Tyson	1 pkg.	3	3	1
nibbles	Swanson	1 pkg.	4	3	7

PREPARED MEAL ITEM	SPECIFICATIONS	BRAND NAME	SERVING SIZE	PROTEIN BLOCKS	CARBOHYDRATE BLOCKS	FAT BLOCKS
Chicken entree, frozen, see also Chicken entree, refrigerated (cont'd)	and noodles	The Budget Gourmet	1 pkg.	3	3	8
	and noodles	Stouffer's Homestyle	1 pkg.	3	2	4
	noodle casserole	Swanson	1 pkg.	2	3	3
	noodle casserole, w/vegetables	Swanson	1 pkg.	3	3	5
	nuggets	Banquet	6 pcs.	2	1	5
	nuggets	Banquet	6 pcs.	2	3	6
	nuggets	Banquet, Homestyle	7 oz.	3	3	7
	nuggets	Country Skillet	10 pcs.	2	2	6
	nuggets	Kid Cuisine Cosmic	1 pkg.	3	5	5
	nuggets	Morton	1 pkg.	2	3	6
	nuggets, mozzarella	Banquet	6 pcs.	2	2	5
	nuggets, Southern	Banquet	6 pcs.	2	2	7
	a l'orange	Lean Cuisine	1 pkg.	3	4	1
	orange glazed	The Budget Gourmet Light & Healthy	1 pkg.	2	6	1

Oriental	Banquet	1 pkg.	2	3	3
Oriental	The Budget Gourmet Light & Healthy	1 pkg.	3	4	2
Oriental	Lean Cuisine	1 pkg.	3	3	2
Oriental	Stouffer's Lunch Express	1 pkg.	2	6	4
Parmesan	Lean Cuisine Café Classics	1 pkg.	3	2	2
parmigiana	Banquet	1 pkg.	2	3	5
parmigiana	Banquet Family Size	5-oz. pc.	2	2	4
parmigiana	Stouffer's Homestyle	1 pkg.	4	3	3
parmigiana	Tyson	1 pkg.	2	3	4
parmigiana	Weight Watchers	1 pkg.	3	4	2
parmigiana, italian style	Banquet	5-oz. pc.	2	2	5
patties, breaded	Banquet	1 pkg.	2	3	7
patties, breaded	Banquet	2 1/2-oz. pc.	1	1	4
patties, breaded	Country Skillet	2 1/2-oz. pc.	1	1	4
patties, breaded	Morton	1 pkg.	2	2	5
patties, breaded	Tyson Thick'n Crispy	2 1/2-oz. pc.	1	1	5
patties, breaded, strips	Swanson	1 pkg.	4	3	6

PREPARED MEAL ITEM	SPECIFICATIONS	BRAND NAME	SERVING SIZE	PROTEIN BLOCKS	CARBOHYDRATE BLOCKS	FAT BLOCKS
Chicken entree, frozen, see also Chicken entree, refrigerated *(cont'd)*	patties, breaded, breast	Tyson	2 1/2-oz. pc.	1	1	4
	patties, breaded, breast, Southern	Tyson	2 1/2-oz. pc.	2	1	4
	patties, breaded, w/cheddar	Tyson Chick'n with Cheddar	1 pc.	2	1	5
	patties, breaded, Southern	Tyson Chick'n Chunks	6 pcs.	1	1	6
	patties, breaded, Southern	Banquet	2 1/3-oz. pc.	1	1	3
	patties, breaded, Southern	Country Skillet	3 1/3-oz. pc.	1	1	4
	in peanut sauce	Lean Cuisine	1 pkg.	3	3	2
	penne pollo	Weight Watchers	1 pkg.	3	4	2
	piccata	Lean Cuisine Café Classics	1 pkg.	2	5	2
	piccata, lemon herb	Smart Ones	1 pkg.	1	3	1
	piccata, w/potato, broccoli	Tyson	1 pkg.	2	2	2
	pie or pot pie	Banquet	1 pkg.	1	4	6
	pie or pot pie	Banquet Family Size	1 pkg.	2	4	10
	pie or pot pie	Empire Kosher	1 pkg.	3	3	7
	pie or pot pie	Lean Cuisine	1 pkg.	3	4	3

pie or pot pie	Marie Callender's	10-oz. pie	2	6	15
pie or pot pie	Marie Callender's	8 1/2-oz. cup	2	5	10
pie or pot pie	Stouffer's	10 oz.	3	4	12
pie or pot pie	Stouffer's	1/2 of 16-oz. pkg.	2	4	12
pie or pot pie	Swanson	1 pkg.	5	5	7
pie or pot pie	Swanson Deluxe	1 pkg.	5	5	7
pie or pot pie	Swanson Hungry Man	1 pkg.	8	7	12
pie or pot pie	Tyson Meat Lovers	9-oz. pie	2	5	13
pie or pot pie	Tyson Meat Lovers	8 1/2-oz. cup	2	5	12
pie or pot pie au gratin	Marie Callender's	10-oz. pie	3	5	6
pie or pot pie au gratin	Marie Callender's	8 1/2-oz. cup	3	4	18
pie or pot pie and broccoli	Marie Callender's	10-oz. pie	3	9	16
pie or pot pie and broccoli	Marie Callender's	8 1/2-oz. cup	3	7	16
pie or pot pie, broccoli and cheese	Tyson	9-oz. pie	3	5	12
pie or pot pie, broccoli and cheese	Tyson	8 1/2-oz. cup	2	5	11

PREPARED MEAL ITEM	SPECIFICATIONS	BRAND NAME	SERVING SIZE	PROTEIN BLOCKS	CARBOHYDRATE BLOCKS	FAT BLOCKS
Chicken entree, frozen, see also Chicken entree, refrigerated (cont'd)	pie or pot pie, and vegetables	Tyson	9-oz. pie	2	5	12
	pie or pot pie, and vegetables	Tyson	8 1/2-oz. cup	2	5	12
	primavera, w/pasta	Banquet	1 pkg.	2	4	4
	primavera, w/pasta	Tyson	1 pkg.	4	5	3
	and rice, stir-fry casserole	Swanson	1 pkg.	1	5	1
	w/rice	Goya Arroz con Pollo	1 pkg.	7	8	9
	roast, glazed	Weight Watchers	1 pkg.	3	3	2
	roasted, herb	Lean Cuisine Café Classics	1 pkg.	2	2	2
	roasted, w/linguini, broccoli	Tyson	1 pkg.	3	2	1
	sesame	Healthy Choice	1 pkg.	2	4	1
	sesame, Shanghai	Healthy Choice	1 pkg.	3	4	2
	stir-fry	Tyson Kit	1 cup	1	3	1
	supreme, w/potato, green beans	Tyson	1 pkg.	2	2	3

	sweet and sour	The Budget Gourmet	1 pkg.	3	6	2
	tikka	Curry Classics Makhanwala	1 pkg.	4	1	11
	and vegetables	Lean Cuisine	1 pkg.	3	3	2
	w/vegetables, garden	Stouffer's Lunch Express	1 pkg.	2	5	4
	walnut, crunchy	Chun King	1 pkg.	3	6	6
	wings, barbeque	Tyson	4 pcs.	3	0	5
	wings, teriyaki	Tyson	4 pcs.	3	0	4
Chicken entree, mix	stir-fry	Tyson	1 cup, prepared	1	2	1
Chicken entree, cutlet, breaded		Perdue	3 1/2-oz pc.	1	2	4
Chicken entree, refrigerated, see also "Chicken, refrigerated or frozen"						
	Italian	Perdue Short Cuts	3 oz.	3	0	1
	lemon pepper	Perdue Short Cuts	3 oz.	3	0	1
	mesquite	Perdue Short Cuts	3 oz.	3	0	1
	nuggets, breaded	Perdue	5 pcs, 3 oz.	1	1	4
	nuggets, breaded and cheese	Perdue	5 pcs., 3 oz.	2	1	5

PREPARED MEAL ITEM	SPECIFICATIONS	BRAND NAME	SERVING SIZE	PROTEIN BLOCKS	CARBOHYDRATE BLOCKS	FAT BLOCKS
Chicken entree, refrigerated, see also "Chicken, refrigerated or frozen" *(cont'd)*	oven roasted	Perdue Short Cuts	3 oz.	3	0	1
	oven roasted, dark meat	Perdue	3 oz.	2	0	4
	oven roasted, white meat	Perdue	3 oz.	3	0	2
	tenderloins, breaded	Perdue	3 oz.	3	1	2
	wings, barbeque	Perdue	3 oz.	2	0	4
	wings, hot and spicy	Perdue	3 oz.	2	0	4
Chicken sandwich, frozen		Hormel Quick Meal	1 pc.	2	5	4
	broccoli and cheddar	Croissant Pockets	1 pc.	2	4	4
	and cheddar w/broccoli	Hot Pockets	1 pc.	2	4	4
	fajita	Lean Pockets	1 pc.	2	4	3
	glazed, supreme	Lean Pockets	1 pc.	1	4	2
	grilled	Hormel Quick Meal	1 pc.	3	4	3
	Parmesan	Lean Pockets	1 pc.	2	4	3
	pastry	Mrs. Paterson's Aussie Pie	1 pc.	2	5	8

Chili, canned, see also "Chili base"						
	Chi-Chi's San Antonio	w/beans	1 cup	3	2	6
	Gebhardt	w/beans	1 cup	2	2	5
	Hormel	w/beans	1 cup	3	2	6
	Hormel	w/beans	7 1/2-oz. can	2	2	4
	Hormel Micro cup	w/beans	1 cont.	2	2	4
	Hormel Micro cup	w/beans	10 1/2-oz. cont.	3	3	6
	Just Rite	w/beans	1 cup	3	2	8
	Libby's	w/beans	1 cup	2	3	9
	Libby's Diner	w/beans	7 3/4 oz.	2	2	7
	Nalley Real Hearty	w/beans	1 cup	3	2	5
	Nalley Thick	w/beans	1 cup	3	2	3
	Old El Paso	w/beans	1 cup	3	1	2
	Van de Kamp's	w/beans	1 cup	3	2	7
	Wolf	w/beans	1 cup	3	2	6
	Nalley Chili Dog	w/beans, beef and hot dogs	1 cup	3	2	4

PREPARED MEAL ITEM	SPECIFICATIONS	BRAND NAME	SERVING SIZE	PROTEIN BLOCKS	CARBOHYDRATE BLOCKS	FAT BLOCKS
Chili, canned, see also "Chili base" *(cont'd)*	w/beans cheddar	Nalley's	1 cup	3	2	4
	w/beans chunky	Hormel	1 cup	2	2	5
	w/beans hot	Hormel	1 cup	3	2	6
	w/beans hot	Hormel/Hormel Micro Cup	7 1/2 oz.	2	2	4
	w/beans jalapeno	Wolf	1 cup	3	2	6
	w/beans jalapeno, hot	Nalley's	1 cup	3	2	3
	w/out beans	Hormel	1 cup	3	1	10
	w/out beans	Hormel	7 1/2-oz. can	3	1	10
	w/out beans	Hormel Micro Cup	1 cont.	3	1	6
	w/out beans	Libby's	1 cup	3	2	12
	w/out beans	Nalley Big Chunk	1 cup	4	1	5
	w/out beans	Wolf	1 cup	3	2	10
	w/out beans, hot	Hormel	1 cup	3	1	10
	w/out beans, jalapeno	Wolf	1 cup	3	2	10
	w/out beans, onion	Nalley Walla Walla	1 cup.	3	2	5
	turkey w/beans	Hormel	1 cup	3	2	1

	Brand	Serving	P	C	F
turkey w/out beans	Hormel	1 cup	3	2	1
vegetarian	Hormel	1 cup	2	3	0
vegetarian	Natural Touch	1 cup	3	1	4
vegetarian	Worthington	1 cup	3	1	5
vegetarian, all varieties except burrito flavor	Health Valley Nonfat	1/2 cup	1	1	0
vegetarian, burrito flavor	Health Valley	1/2 cup	1	1	0
w/macaroni	Hormel Chili Mac	7 1/2-oz. can	2	2	3
w/macaroni	Hormel Chili Mac Micro Cup	1 cont.	2	2	3
Chili freeze-dried w/beef, beans	Mountain House	1 cup	2	2	1
w/beef, macaroni	Mountain House	1 cup	2	3	2
Chili frozen w/beans	Stouffer's Entree	1 pkg.	2	2	3
w/cornbread	Marie Callender's Dinner	1 pkg.	2	4	4
three bean	Lean Cuisine Entree	1 pkg.	1	3	2
vegetarian	Tabatchnik Side Dish	1 pkg.	2	2	2
Chimichanga, frozen beef	Old El Paso	4 1/2-oz. pc.	1	4	7
beefsteak and bean	Don Miguel	7 oz.	2	6	4

PREPARED MEAL ITEM	SPECIFICATIONS	BRAND NAME	SERVING SIZE	PROTEIN BLOCKS	CARBOHYDRATE BLOCKS	FAT BLOCKS
Chimichanga, frozen *(cont'd)*	chicken	Don Miguel	7 oz.	2	5	4
	chicken	Old El Paso	4 1/2-oz. pc.	2	4	5
Chimichanga dinner, frozen	beef	Chi-Chi's	15 oz.	4	7	9
	chicken	Chi-Chi's	15 oz.	3	7	8
Chimichanga entree	frozen	Banquet	9 1/2 oz.	2	5	3
Egg breakfast, freeze-dried	w/bacon	Mountain House	1/2 cup	2	1	3
	w/bacon, precooked	Mountain House	1/2 cup	1	1	2
	omelet, cheese	Mountain House	1/2 cup	2	1	4
	omelet, ham-cheese	Weight Watchers	1 pkg.	2	3	2
Egg breakfast, frozen, see also specific listings	patty, egg, w/Canadian bacon	Swanson Great Starts	1 pkg.	1	3	2
	patty, egg, w/pork and turkey	Swanson Great Starts	1 pkg.	2	3	3

Egg breakfast sandwich, frozen	scrambled	Swanson Great Starts Egg Product	1 pkg.	3	2	4
	scrambled	Swanson Great Starts Low Fat	1 pkg.	3	2	4
	scrambled and bacon	Swanson Great Starts	1 pkg.	4	2	6
	scrambled w/homefries	Swanson Great Starts	1 pkg.	3	1	4
	scrambled and sausage	Swanson Great Starts	1 pkg.	6	2	9
	w/cheese	Swanson Great Starts	1 pkg.	4	4	6
	muffin	Weight Watchers	1 pkg.	2	3	2
	muffin w/bacon and cheese	Swanson Great Starts	1 pkg.	3	3	5
	muffin w/Canadian bacon and cheese	Hormel Quick Meal	1 pkg.	2	3	3
	muffin w/sausage and cheese	Hormel Quick Meal	1 pkg.	2	3	8
	omelet	Weight Watchers Classic	1 pkg.	2	3	2
Eggplant entree, frozen	cutlets	Celentano	5 oz.	1	2	8
	parmigiana	Celentano	10-oz. pkg.	2	1	9
	parmigiana	Celentano 14 oz.	1/2 pkg.	2	1	7
	parmigiana	Celentano Value Pack	8-oz. cup	1	1	8

PREPARED MEAL ITEM	SPECIFICATIONS	BRAND NAME	SERVING SIZE	PROTEIN BLOCKS	CARBOHYDRATE BLOCKS	FAT BLOCKS
Eggplant entree, frozen *(cont'd)*	parmigiana	Mrs. Paul's	1/2 cup	3	2	5
	rollettes	Celentano	10 oz.	1	2	7
	rollettes	Celentano Great Choice	10 oz.	2	4	5
Enchilada, canned		Gebhardt	2 pcs.	1	2	6
Enchilada, dinner, frozen		Amy's	1 pkg.	1	4	3
		Chi-Chi's Baja	1 pkg.	4	8	6
	beef	Healthy Choice, Rio Grande	1 pkg.	2	0	3
	beef	Patio	1 pkg.	2	5	3
	beef	Patio Chili 'n Beans Large	2 pcs.	2	3	2
	beef	Swanson	1 pkg.	4	6	6
	beef, chili sauce w/	Banquet Family	1 pc.	1	2	5
	beef and cheese	Patio Chili 'n Beans	2 pcs.	2	3	2
	cheese	Patio	1 pkg.	2	5	3
	chicken	Chi-Chi's Suprema	1 pkg.	3	7	8
	chicken	Healthy Choice Suprema	1 pkg.	2	6	3
	chicken	Patio	1 pkg.	2	5	3

Enchilada entree, frozen	beef	Banquet	1 pkg.	2	5	4
	beef	Patio Family	2 pcs.	1	3	2
	beef and tamale, chili gravy w/	Morton	1 pkg.	1	4	2
	black bean	Amy's Family	4 1/2 oz.	1	2	1
	black bean and vegetable	Amy's Family	5 oz.	1	2	1
	cheese	Amy's	1 pkg.	2	2	3
	cheese	Amy's Family	4 1/3 oz.	1	1	3
	cheese	Banquet	1 pkg.	2	5	2
	cheese	Patio Family	2 pcs.	1	2	1
	cheese and rice	Stouffer's	1 pkg.	2	5	5
	chicken	Banquet	1 pkg.	2	5	3
	chicken, nacho grande	Weight Watchers	1 pkg.	2	4	3
	chicken and rice	Stouffer's	1 pkg.	2	5	5
	chicken Suiza	Healthy Choice	1 pkg.	2	4	1
	chicken Suiza	Weight Watchers	1 pkg.	2	3	3
	chicken Suiza, w/rice	Lean Cuisine	1 pkg.	2	5	2

PREPARED MEAL ITEM	SPECIFICATIONS	BRAND NAME	SERVING SIZE	PROTEIN BLOCKS	CARBOHYDRATE BLOCKS	FAT BLOCKS
Fajita, canned	beef	Nalley Superba	1 cup	2	2	2
	chicken	Nalley Superba	1 cup	2	2	2
Fajita entree, frozen	beef	Tyson Kit	3 1/2-oz. fajita	1	2	1
	chicken	Healthy Choice Fiesta	7 oz.	3	3	1
	chicken	Tyson Kit	3 1/2-oz. fajita	1	2	1
Fettuccine entree, frozen	Alfredo	Banquet	1 pkg.	2	4	6
	Alfredo	Healthy Choice	1 pkg.	2	4	2
	Alfredo	Lean Cuisine	1 pkg.	2	4	2
	Alfredo	Marie Callender's	1 cup	1	3	7
	Alfredo	Stouffer's	1 pkg.	2	4	13
	Alfredo, w/broccoli	Weight Watchers	1 pkg.	1	3	2
	Alfredo w/four cheeses	The Budget Gourmet	1 pkg.	3	5	8
	w/broccoli and chicken	Marie Callender's	1 cup	3	3	9
	primavera	Lean Cuisine	1 pkg.	2	3	3
	primavera	Marie Callender's	1 cup	1	3	6

Fish dinner, frozen see also specific fish listings	primavera	Stouffer's Lunch Express	1 pkg.	2	3	8
	battered portions w/chips	Swanson	1 pkg.	4	6	7
Fish entree, frozen, see also specific fish listings	breaded sticks	Swanson Budget	1 pkg.	2	5	4
		Van de Kamp's Fish'n Fries	6 1/2 oz.	2	4	6
	baked, w/shells	Lean Cuisine	9 oz.	3	3	3
	cakes	Mrs. Paul's	2 pcs.	2	2	3
	and chips	Swanson	1 pkg.	3	4	4
	fillets, battered	Gorton's	2 pcs.	1	2	6
	fillets, battered	Mrs. Paul's	1 pc.	2	1	4
	fillets, battered	Mrs. Paul's Crunchy	2 pcs.	3	2	4
	fillets, battered	Van de Kamp's	1 pc.	1	1	4
	fillets, battered, lemon pepper	Gorton's	2 pcs.	1	2	5

PREPARED MEAL ITEM	SPECIFICATIONS	BRAND NAME	SERVING SIZE	PROTEIN BLOCKS	CARBOHYDRATE BLOCKS	FAT BLOCKS
Fish entree, frozen, see also specific fish listings *(cont'd)*	fillets, breaded	Gorton's Crunchy	2 pcs.	2	2	6
	fillets, breaded	Mrs. Paul's	2 pcs.	3	2	4
	fillets, breaded	Mrs. Paul's Healthy Treasures	1 pc.	1	2	1
	fillets, breaded	Van de Kamp's	2 pcs.	2	2	6
	fillets, breaded	Van de Kamp's Crisp and Healthy	2 pcs.	2	2	1
	fillets, breaded, garlic and herb	Gorton's Crunchy	2 pcs.	1	2	5
	fillets, breaded, hot and spicy	Gorton's Crunchy	2 pcs.	1	2	5
	fillets, breaded, potato	Gorton's	2 pcs.	2	2	7
	fillets, breaded, Southern fried	Gorton's Crunchy	2 pcs.	2	2	5
	fillets, grilled, Italian herb	Gorton's	1 pc.	3	0	2
	fillets, grilled, lemon pepper	Gorton's	1 pc.	2	0	2
	fillets, in sauce	Mrs. Paul's Kitchen	1 pc.	1	0	2

fillets, in sauce, lemon pepper	Healthy Choice	11 oz.	2	4	2
grilled, w/vegetables	Lean Cuisine Café Classics	9 oz.	2	1	2
w/macaroni and cheese	Stouffer's Homestyle	9 oz.	3	4	7
w/macaroni and cheese	Swanson	1 pkg.	3	4	5
nuggets	Van de Kamp's	8 pcs.	2	2	6
portions, battered	Gorton's	1 pc.	1	1	3
portions, battered	Mrs. Paul's	2 pcs.	4	2	6
portions, battered	Van de Kamp's	2 pcs.	2	3	7
portions, breaded	Mrs. Paul's	2 pcs.	2	2	3
portions, breaded	Van de Kamp's	3 pcs.	2	3	7
shapes, breaded	Mrs. Paul's Sea Pals	5 pcs.	2	2	3
sticks	Kid Cuisine Funtastic	1 pkg.	2	6	4
sticks	Swanson Fun Feast Frenzied	1 pkg.	3	5	5
sticks, battered	Gorton's	5 pcs.	1	2	7
sticks, battered	Mrs. Paul's	6 pcs.	3	1	4
sticks, battered	Mrs. Paul's Crispy Crunchy	6 pcs.	2	2	5

PREPARED MEAL ITEM	SPECIFICATIONS	BRAND NAME	SERVING SIZE	PROTEIN BLOCKS	CARBOHYDRATE BLOCKS	FAT BLOCKS
Fish entree, frozen, see also specific fish listings (cont'd)	sticks, breaded	Gorton's Crunchy	6 pcs.	2	2	5
	sticks, breaded	Mrs. Paul's	6 pcs.	2	2	4
	sticks, breaded	Mrs. Paul's Crispy Crunchy	5 pcs.	2	2	5
	sticks, breaded	Gorton's Value Pack	6 pcs.	1	2	4
	sticks, breaded	Van de Kamp's	6 pcs.	2	3	6
	sticks, breaded	Van de Kamp's Snack/Value Pack	6 pcs.	2	2	5
	sticks, breaded	Van de Kamp's Crisp and Healthy	6 pcs.	2	3	1
	sticks, breaded, mini	Mrs. Paul's	12 pcs.	2	2	4
	sticks, breaded, mini	Van de Kamp's	13 pcs.	2	2	5
	sticks, breaded, potato	Gorton's	6 pcs.	1	2	5
Fish sandwich	fillet, frozen	Hormel Quick Meal	1 pc.	2	5	5
	fillet, frozen, w/cheese	Mrs. Paul's	1 pc.	3	4	5
Flounder entree, fillets, frozen	battered	Mrs. Paul's Crunchy	2 pcs.	3	2	5
	breaded	Mrs. Paul's Premium	1 pc.	3	2	4

breaded		Van de Kamp's Light	1 pkg.	2	2	4
Frankfurter sandwich, frozen		Hormel Quick Meal Jumbo Dog	1 pc.	2	3	7
	bagel wrapped	Boar's Head Bagel Dog	1 pc.	2	0	9
	bagel wrapped	Hebrew National Bagel Dog	1 pc.	2	5	6
	on bun	Swanson Fun Feast	1 pc.	3	5	4
	w/cheese	Hormel Quick Meal Cheesey Dog	1 pc.	1	3	6
	chili w/cheese	Hormel Quick Meal	1 pc.	2	3	7
	corn dog	Hormel/Hormel Quick Meal	1 pc.	1	3	4
	corn dog, mini	Hormel Quick Meal	1 pc.	1	2	5
French toast, frozen		Aunt Jemima	2 pcs.	1	4	2
		Downyflake	2 pcs.	1	5	2
	cinnamon swirl	Aunt Jemima	2 pcs.	1	4	2
	cinnamon swirl	Downyflake	2 pcs.	1	5	2
French toast breakfast, frozen	cinnamon swirl	Swanson Great Starts	2 pcs.	6	4	9
	w/sausage	Swanson Great Starts	2 pcs.	6	3	9
	sticks, mini	Swanson Kids Breakfast	2 pcs.	3	4	5

PREPARED MEAL ITEM	SPECIFICATIONS	BRAND NAME	SERVING SIZE	PROTEIN BLOCKS	CARBOHYDRATE BLOCKS	FAT BLOCKS
Haddock entree, frozen	battered	Mrs. Paul's Crunchy	2 pcs.	3	3	4
	battered	Van de Kamp's	2 pcs.	2	2	5
	breaded	Mrs. Paul's	1 pc.	2	2	4
	breaded	Van de Kamp's	2 pcs.	2	2	6
	breaded	Van de Kamp's Light	1 pc.	2	2	3
Halibut entree	frozen, battered	Van de Kamp's	3 pcs.	2	2	7
Ham and asparagus	frozen, baked	Stouffer's	9 1/2 oz.	2	3	12
Ham and asparagus au gratin	frozen	The Budget Gourmet Light & Healthy	9 oz.	2	3	4
Ham and cheese sandwich	frozen	Croissant Pockets	1 pc.	2	4	6
	frozen	Hormel Quick Meal	1 pc.	3	5	3
	frozen	Hot Pockets	1 pc.	2	4	5
Herring salad		Vita	1/4 cup	1	2	1
Lamb curry entree	frozen	Curry Classics	10 oz.	5	1	10

		Serving			
Lasagna entree, canned	Hormel	7 1/2-oz. can	1	3	5
	Hormel Micro Cup	7 1/2 oz.	1	3	5
	Libby's Diner	7 3/4 oz.	1	2	2
	Nalley's	1 cup	2	3	2
and beef	Nalley's	7 1/2-oz. can	1	2	2
cheese, three	Hormel Micro Cup	10 1/2 oz.	2	3	6
	Nalley's	7 1/2-oz. can	2	2	2
Italian	Top Shelf	10 oz.	3	3	5
Lasagna entree, freeze dried	Mountain House	1 cup	2	2	3
Lasagna entree, frozen	Celentano	1 pkg.	3	5	5
	Celentano	1/2 of 14-oz. pkg.	2	3	3
	Celentano 25 oz.	1 cup	3	2	6
	Celentano Great Choice	1 pkg.	3	4	1
	Celentano Value Pack	1 cup	2	4	4
	Healthy Choice Roma	1 pkg.	4	6	2
cheese	Lean Cuisine Classic	1 pkg.	3	4	2
cheese casserole	Lean Cuisine Lunch Express	1 pkg.	2	4	2

PREPARED MEAL ITEM	SPECIFICATIONS	BRAND NAME	SERVING SIZE	PROTEIN BLOCKS	CARBOHYDRATE BLOCKS	FAT BLOCKS
Lasagna entree, frozen *(cont'd)*	cheese, w/chicken scaloppini	Lean Cuisine Café Classics	1 pkg.	3	3	3
	cheese, four	Stouffer's	1 pkg.	3	4	6
	cheese, italian	Weight Watchers	1 pkg.	3	4	3
	cheese, three	The Budget Gourmet	1 pkg.	3	4	5
	extra cheese	Marie Callender's	1 cup	2	3	5
	Florentine	Smart Ones	1 pkg.	1	3	1
	garden	Weight Watchers	1 pkg.	2	3	2
	w/meat sauce	Banquet	1 pkg.	2	4	3
	w/meat sauce	Banquet Bake at Home	8-oz. cup	2	3	2
	w/meat sauce	Banquet Family	1 cup	2	0	3
	w/meat sauce	The Budget Gourmet Light and Healthy	1 pkg.	2	3	2
	w/meat sauce	Lean Cuisine	1 pkg.	3	3	3
	w/meat sauce	Marie Callender's	7 oz.	2	3	6

w/meat sauce	Stouffer's	1 pkg.	4	3	4
w/meat sauce	Stouffer's	21-oz. pkg.	9	6	9
w/meat sauce	Stouffer's Lunch Express	1 pkg.	3	4	3
w/meat sauce	Swanson	1 pkg.	3	4	5
w/meat sauce	Weight Watchers	1 pkg.	2	4	2
w/meat sauce	Swanson	1 pkg.	2	4	3
w/meat sauce, casserole	Celentano Great Choice	1 pkg.	2	3	2
primavera	Celentano Selects	1 pkg.	2	3	1
primavera	The Budget Gourmet	1 pkg.	3	4	7
sausage, Italian	Amy's Family	7 oz.	1	3	3
vegetable	Banquet	1 pkg.	2	4	2
vegetable	The Budget Gourmet Light and Healthy	1 pkg.	2	3	3
vegetable	Lean Cuisine	1 pkg.	2	4	2
vegetable	Stouffer's	1 pkg.	3	4	8
vegetable	Stouffer's	96-oz. pkg.	24	36	72
vegetable w/cheese	Amy's	1 pkg.	2	4	3
vegetable, cheesy	Swanson	1 pkg.	3	4	4

PREPARED MEAL ITEM	SPECIFICATIONS	BRAND NAME	SERVING SIZE	PROTEIN BLOCKS	CARBOHYDRATE BLOCKS	FAT BLOCKS
Lasagna entree, frozen *(cont'd)*	vegetable, tofu	Amy's	1 pkg.	3	4	3
Linguine entree, frozen	w/shrimp and clams	The Budget Gourmet Light & Healthy	1 pkg.	2	4	3
	w/shrimp and clams, marinara	The Budget Gourmet	1 pkg.	2	4	4
	w/tomato sauce and sausage	The Budget Gourmet	1 pkg.	2	4	5
Lunch combinations	bologna/American	Lunchables	1 pkg.	2	2	12
	bologna/wild cherry	Lunchables	1 pkg.	2	7	9
	chicken/turkey deluxe	Lunchables	1 pkg.	3	3	8
	ham/cheddar	Lunchables	1 pkg.	3	2	7
	ham/Swiss	Lunchables	1 pkg.	3	2	7
	ham/fruit punch	Lunchables	1 pkg.	2	6	7
	ham/fruit punch, low fat	Lunchables	1 pkg.	2	6	3
	ham/Surfer Cooler	Lunchables	1 pkg.	3	6	3
	pizza, mozzarella, cheddar	Lunchables	1 pkg.	3	3	5

pizza, mozzarella, fruit punch	Lunchables	1 pkg.	3	7	6
pizza/pepperoni, mozzarella	Lunchables	1 pkg.	2	3	5
pizza/pepperoni, orange	Lunchables	1 pkg.	3	7	6
salami/American	Lunchables	1 pkg.	3	2	10
turkey/cheddar	Lunchables	1 pkg.	3	2	7
turkey/ham	Lunchables	1 pkg.	3	3	7
turkey/Monterey Jack	Lunchables	1 pkg.	3	2	7
turkey/Pacific Cooler	Lunchables	1 pkg.	2	6	7
turkey/Pacific Cooler, low fat	Lunchables	1 pkg.	2	6	3
turkey/Surfer Cooler	Lunchables	1 pkg.	2	7	5
Macaroni dinner, and cheese, frozen	Swanson Budget	1 pkg.	2	4	4
Macaroni entree, canned, and beef	Kid's Kitchen Beefy	7 1/2 oz.	2	2	2
and beef	Kid's Kitchen Cheezy Mac & Beef	7 1/2 oz.	2	4	2
and beef	Libby's Diner	7 3/4 oz.	1	3	3
and cheese	Chef Boyardee Bowl	7 1/2 oz.	1	3	0
and cheese	Franco-American	1 cup	2	3	2

PREPARED MEAL ITEM	SPECIFICATIONS	BRAND NAME	SERVING SIZE	PROTEIN BLOCKS	CARBOHYDRATE BLOCKS	FAT BLOCKS
Macaroni entree, canned (cont'd)	and cheese	Hormel Micro Cup	7 1/2 oz.	2	3	4
	and cheese	Libby's Diner	7 3/4 oz.	2	3	7
	and cheese	Kid's Kitchen	7 1/2 oz.	2	3	4
Macaroni entree, frozen	and beef	Banquet Bake at Home	8-oz. cup	2	3	2
	and beef	Kid Cuisine Riproaring	1 pkg.	2	6	5
	and beef	Lean Cuisine	1 pkg.	2	4	3
	and beef	Marie Callender's	1 pkg.	2	4	4
	and beef	Nalley's	1 pkg.	1	2	5
	and beef	Stouffer's	1 pkg.	3	4	7
	and beef	Weight Watchers	1 pkg.	2	2	2
	and beef, casserole	Healthy Choice	1 pkg.	2	3	3
	and beef, casserole	Swanson	1 pkg.	1	4	2
	broccoli	Swanson Mac & More	1 pkg.	2	3	3
	and cheese	Amy's	1 pkg.	3	6	3
	and cheese	Banquet	1 pkg.	2	5	4

and cheese	Banquet Bake at Home	8 oz.	2	4	3
and cheese	Banquet Family	1 cup	1	3	2
and cheese	The Budget Gourmet Homestyle	1 pkg.	2	4	7
and cheese	The Budget Gourmet Side Dish	6 oz.	2	3	4
and cheese	Healthy Choice	1 pkg.	2	4	1
and cheese	Kid Cuisine Magical	1 pkg.	1	7	4
and cheese	Lean Cuisine	1 pkg.	2	4	2
and cheese	Marie Callender's	1 pkg.	3	5	6
and cheese	Morton	1 pkg.	1	4	1
and cheese	Morton 16/28 oz.	1 cup	1	4	1
and cheese	Stouffer's	1/2 of 12-oz. pkg.	2	3	6
and cheese	Stouffer's	1 pkg.	10	15	25
and cheese	Swanson Entree	1 pkg.	2	4	3
and cheese	Swanson Entree	1 cup	2	4	3
and cheese	Swanson Mac & More Classic	1 pkg.	2	3	3
and cheese	Tabatchnik Side Dish	1 pkg.	2	3	4
and cheese	Weight Watchers	1 pkg.	2	4	2

PREPARED MEAL ITEM	SPECIFICATIONS	BRAND NAME	SERVING SIZE	PROTEIN BLOCKS	CARBOHYDRATE BLOCKS	FAT BLOCKS
Macaroni entree, frozen *(cont'd)*	and cheese bake casserole, 3 cheese	Swanson	1 pkg.	3	6	5
	and cheese, and broccoli	Lean Cuisine Lunch Express	1 pkg.	2	3	2
	and cheese, w/cheddar and Parmesan	The Budget Gourmet Light & Healthy	1 pkg.	1	5	3
	and cheese, cheddar, white	Swanson Mac & More	1 pkg.	2	3	2
	and cheese, pie	Banquet	1 pkg.	1	4	1
	and cheese, salsa	Swanson Mac & More	1 pkg.	2	3	3
	Italiano	Swanson Mac & More	1 pkg.	1	3	2
	soy cheeze	Amy's	1 pkg.	2	4	5
Manicotti entree, frozen	cheese	Celentano	1 pkg.	3	4	7
	cheese	Celentano	14-oz. pkg.	4	4	10
	cheese	Celentano Great Choice	1 pkg.	2	4	1
	cheese	Celentano Value Pack	2 pcs., 8 oz.	2	2	5
	cheese	Stouffer's	1 pkg.	3	3	5

			P	C	F
cheese	Weight Watchers	1 pkg.	2	3	2
cheese, w/meat sauce	The Budget Gourmet	1 pkg.	3	4	7
cheese, three cheese	Healthy Choice	1 pkg.	2	4	3
Florentine	Celentano	1 pkg.	2	3	2
Florentine	Celentano Great Choice	1 pkg.	2	3	2
Meat loaf dinner, frozen	Banquet	1 pkg.	4	4	13
	Healthy Choice	1 pkg.	2	4	3
	Marie Callender's	1 pkg.	3	4	10
	Swanson	1 pkg.	4	4	5
	Swanson Budget	1 pkg.	4	3	6
	Swanson Hungry Man	1 pkg.	6	7	9
Meat loaf entree, frozen	Banquet Homestyle	1 pkg.	2	2	6
w/whipped potato	Lean Cuisine	1 pkg.	3	2	2
	Stouffer's Homestyle	1 pkg.	3	2	8
tomato sauce,	Morton	1 pkg.	1	2	4
w/sauce and vegetables	Swanson	1 pkg.	3	1	4
Meatball entree, frozen					
kofta curry	Deep	1 pkg.	1	2	5
Swedish	The Budget Gourmet	1 pkg.	3	4	11

PREPARED MEAL ITEM	SPECIFICATIONS	BRAND NAME	SERVING SIZE	PROTEIN BLOCKS	CARBOHYDRATE BLOCKS	FAT BLOCKS
Meatball entree,	Swedish	Healthy Choice	1 pkg.	3	4	3
frozen *(cont'd)*	Swedish	Stouffer's	1 pkg.	3	4	8
	Swedish	Weight Watchers	1 pkg.	3	3	3
	Swedish, w/broccoli	Stouffer's Lunch Express	1 pkg.	2	3	6
	Swedish, w/pasta	Lean Cuisine	1 pkg.	3	3	3
	Swedish, w/pasta	Stouffer's Lunch Express	1 pkg.	3	4	11
Meatball stew, canned		Dinty Moore	1 cup	2	2	5
		Dinty Moore Cup	7 1/2 oz.	2	2	5
		Patio	1 pkg.	2	5	5
Mexican dinners, frozen,						
see also specific listings						
		Patio Fiesta	1 pkg.	2	4	3
		Patio Ranchera	1 pkg.	2	5	5
	style	Banquet	1 pkg.	4	9	11
	style	Swanson Budget	1 pkg.	4	5	5
	style	Swanson Hungry Man	1 pkg.	8	8	12
	style, combination	Swanson	1 pkg.	4	5	6

			1 pkg.	2	5	4
Mexican entree, frozen, see also specific listings		Banquet				
	combination	Banquet	1 pkg.	2	5	4
Noodle entree, canned	w/beef	Hunt's Homestyle	1 cup	1	2	1
	w/beef	La Choy Bi-Pack	1 cup	2	2	0
	w/chicken	Dinty Moore	7 1/2 oz.	1	2	3
	w/chicken	Hormel Micro Cup	7 1/2 oz.	1	2	3
	w/chicken	Hormel Micro Cup	10 1/2 oz.	2	3	4
	w/chicken	La Choy Bi-Pack	1 cup	2	2	1
	w/chicken	Nalley Dinner	1 cup	1	2	2
	w/chicken	Nalley Dinner	7 1/2 oz.	1	2	1
	w/chicken, cacciatore or regular	Hunt's Homestyle	1 cup	2	2	2
	w/chicken, w/mushrooms	Hunt's Homestyle	1 cup	1	3	2
	w/franks	Van de Kamp's Noodle Weenee	1 can	1	4	3
	rings	Kid's Kitchen	7 1/2 oz.	2	2	2
	sweet and sour, w/chicken	La Choy Entree	1 cup	1	4	1

PREPARED MEAL ITEM	SPECIFICATIONS	BRAND NAME	SERVING SIZE	PROTEIN BLOCKS	CARBOHYDRATE BLOCKS	FAT BLOCKS
Noodle entree, canned (cont'd)	w/vegetables	La Choy Entree	1 cup	1	3	0
	w/vegetables and beef	La Choy Entree	1 cup	1	3	1
	w/vegetables and chicken	La Choy Entree	1 cup	1	3	1
Noodle entree, frozen	and beef	Banquet Family	1 pkg.	2	2	1
	and chicken	Banquet Bake at Home	1 pkg.	1	2	3
	and chicken, escalloped	Marie Callender's	6 1/2 oz.	1	2	5
	escalloped, and turkey	The Budget Gourmet	1 pkg.	3	5	7
	kung pao, and vegetables	Weight Watchers	1 pkg.	1	3	3
	Romanoff	Stouffer's	1 pkg.	3	5	8
Pancake breakfast, frozen		Swanson Kids Breakfast Blast Mini	1 pkg.	2	6	3
	w/bacon	Swanson Great Starts	1 pkg.	4	5	7
	w/sausage	Swanson Great Starts	1 pkg.	5	5	8
	silver dollar, eggs and	Swanson Great Starts	1 pkg.	3	2	5
	silver dollar, and sausage	Swanson Great Starts	1 pkg.	4	3	6

Food	Brand	Serving	P	C	F
Pasta dishes, frozen, see also "Pasta entree, frozen"					
Alfredo	Green Giant Pasta Accents	2 cups	1	2	3
Alfredo, w/broccoli	The Budget Gourmet Side Dish	6 oz.	1	2	4
cheddar, creamy	Green Giant Pasta Accents	2 1/3 cups	1	4	3
cheddar, white	Green Giant Pasta Accents	1 3/4 cups	1	4	4
garden herb	Green Giant Pasta Accents	2 cups	1	3	2
garlic	Green Giant Pasta Accents	2 cups	1	3	3
Florentine	Green Giant Pasta Accents	2 cups	2	4	3
primavera	Green Giant Pasta Accents	2 1/4 cups	2	4	4
spirals, and chicken	Libby's Diner	7 3/4 oz.	1	1	1
Pasta entree, canned, see also specific listings					
twists	Franco-American	1 cup	1	4	2
primavera	Mountain House	1 cup	1	3	2
Pasta entree, freeze-dried					
Roma	Alpine Aire	1 1/2 cups	3	5	0

PREPARED MEAL ITEM	SPECIFICATIONS	BRAND NAME	SERVING SIZE	PROTEIN BLOCKS	CARBOHYDRATE BLOCKS	FAT BLOCKS
Pasta entree, frozen, see also "Pasta dishes, frozen" and specific pasta listings	cheddar bake w/	Lean Cuisine	1 pkg.	2	3	2
	cheddar and broccoli	Banquet	1 pkg.	2	5	4
	and chicken marinara	Lean Cuisine Lunch Express	1 pkg.	2	4	2
	marinara twist	Lean Cuisine	1 pkg.	1	4	1
	primavera, w/chicken	Marie Callender's	1 cup	2	2	6
	rings	Swanson Fun Feast "Razzlin'"	1 pkg.	3	6	4
	sausage and peppers	Banquet	1 pkg.	2	4	4
	and spinach Romano	Weight Watchers	1 pkg.	2	3	3
	w/tomato basil sauce	Weight Watchers	1 pkg.	2	3	3
	and tuna casserole	Lean Cuisine Lunch Express	1 pkg.	3	4	2
	and turkey Dijon	Lean Cuisine Lunch Express	1 pkg.	2	3	2
	vegetable Italiano	Healthy Choice	1 pkg.	1	5	0
	wheels and cheese	Swanson Fun Feast	1 pkg.	2	6	4

Penne entree, canned	wide ribbon w/ricotta	The Budget Gourmet	1 pkg.	2	6	2
	in meat sauce	Franco-American	1 cup	1	6	0
Penne entree, frozen	w/sausage	The Budget Gourmet Light & Healthy	1 pkg.	2	7	1
	spicy and ricotta	Weight Watchers	1 pkg.	2	6	0
	w/sun-dried tomato	Weight Watchers	1 pkg.	2	6	1
Pepper "steak" entree, vegetarian	frozen	Hain	10 oz.	4	4	2
Pepperoni bagel sandwich	frozen	Hormel Quick Meal	1 pc.	2	4	5
Pierogi, frozen or refrigerated	potato cheese	Empire Kosher	4 oz.	2	4	1
	potato onion	Empire Kosher	4 oz.	1	4	0
	potato onion	Giorgio	3 pcs.	1	4	1
Pizza, frozen	artichoke heart	Wolfgang Puck	1 pie	2	3	6
	Canadian bacon	Tombstone Original 12"	1 pie	12	16	20
	Canadian bacon	Totino's Party	1 pie	2	3	5
	Canadian bacon	Jeno's Crisp 'n Tasty	1 pie	2	5	6

PREPARED MEAL ITEM	SPECIFICATIONS	BRAND NAME	SERVING SIZE	PROTEIN BLOCKS	CARBOHYDRATE BLOCKS	FAT BLOCKS
Pizza, frozen *(cont'd)*	Canadian bacon	Celentano Thick Crust	1/2 pie	3	6	4
	cheese	Celeste Large	1/4 pie	2	3	5
	cheese	Celeste for One	1 pie	3	6	8
	cheese	Empire Kosher 3 Pack	1 pie	1	2	3
	cheese	Empire Kosher 10 oz.	1/2 pie	3	4	4
	cheese	Jeno's Crisp 'n Tasty	1 pie	3	5	6
	cheese	Jeno's Microwave	1 pie	1	3	4
	cheese	Swanson Fun Feast	1 pie	2	6	3
	cheese	Tombstone For One 1/2 Less Fat	1 pie	3	5	3
	cheese	Totino's Microwave	1 pie	1	3	4
	cheese	Totino's Party	1/2 pie	2	3	5
	cheese	Totino's Party Family Size	1/3 pie	2	4	5
	cheese, extra	Marie Callender's	1/2 pie	2	3	8
	cheese, extra	Tombstone Original 9"	1/2 pie	3	4	6
	cheese, extra	Tombstone Original 12"	1/4 pie	3	4	6
	cheese, extra	Tombstone For One	1 pie	4	4	10

cheese, extra	Weight Watchers	1 pie	3	5	4
cheese, three	Pappalo's Deep Dish	1/4 pie	3	5	4
cheese, three	Pappalo's Deep Dish for One	1 pie	4	6	7
cheese, three	Pappalo's For One	1 pie	4	5	7
cheese, three	Pappalo's 9"	1/2 pie	3	5	5
cheese, three	Pappalo's 12"	1/4 pie	3	4	4
cheese, three	Totino's Select	1/3 pie	2	3	5
cheese, three, Italian	Tombstone Thin crust	1/4 pie	3	3	7
cheese, four	Celeste for One	1 pie	4	5	10
cheese, four	Tombstone Special Order 12"	1/5 pie	3	4	6
cheese, four	Wolfgang Puck	1/2 pie	2	4	5
cheese, four, hot and zesty	Celeste For One	1 pie	3	5	9
cheese, four, zesty	Celeste Large	1/4 pie	2	3	5
cheese, two, w/Canadian bacon	Totino's Select	1/3 pie	2	3	5
cheese, two, w/pepperoni	Totino's Select	1/3 pie	2	3	7
cheese, two, w/sausage	Totino's Select	1/3 pie	2	3	6
chicken and broccoli	Marie Callender's	1/2 pie	3	4	5

PREPARED MEAL ITEM	SPECIFICATIONS	BRAND NAME	SERVING SIZE	PROTEIN BLOCKS	CARBOHYDRATE BLOCKS	FAT BLOCKS
Pizza, frozen *(cont'd)*	combination	Jeno's Microwave	1 pie	2	3	6
	combination	Jeno's Crisp 'n Tasty	1 pie	2	5	9
	combination	Totino's Microwave	1 pie	2	3	6
	combination	Totino's Party	1/2 pie	2	4	7
	combination	Totino's Party Family	1/4 pie	2	3	5
	combination	Weight Watchers	1 pie	3	5	4
	deluxe	Celeste Large	1/4 pie	2	3	6
	deluxe	Celeste for One	1 pie	3	5	10
	deluxe	Marie Callender's	1/2 pie	2	3	8
	deluxe	Tombstone Original 9"	1/3 pie	2	3	5
	deluxe	Tombstone Original 12"	1/4 pie	2	3	5
	hamburger	Jeno's Crisp 'n Tasty	1 pie	3	5	8
	hamburger	Tombstone Original 9"	1/3 pie	2	3	5
	hamburger	Tombstone Original 12"	1/5 pie	2	3	5
	hamburger	Totino's Party	1/2 pie	2	3	6
	Italiano, zesty	Totino's Party	1/2 pie	2	4	7

w/meat	Celeste Suprema for One	1 pie	4	5	10
w/meat	Celeste Suprema, Large	1/5 pie	2	3	5
meat, five	Marie Callender's	1/2 pie	2	4	5
meat, four	Tombstone Special Order 9"	1/3 pie	3	4	7
meat, four	Tombstone Special Order 12"	1/6 pie	2	3	6
meat, four, combo, Italian	Tombstone Thin Crust	1/4 pie	3	3	8
meat, three	Jeno's Crisp 'n Tasty	1 pie	3	5	9
meat, three	Totino's Party	1/2 pie	2	3	6
Mexican style, supreme taco	Tombstone Thin Crust	1/4 pie	2	3	8
Mexican style, zesty	Totino's Microwave	1 pie	1	3	5
Mexican style, zesty	Totino's Party	1/2 pie	2	4	6
pepperoni	Celeste Large	1/4 pie	2	3	7
pepperoni	Celeste Pizza for One	1 pie	3	5	9
pepperoni	Hormel Quick Meal	1 pie	3	5	5
pepperoni	Jeno's Microwave	1 pie	1	3	5
pepperoni	Jeno's Crisp 'n Tasty	1 pie	2	5	9
pepperoni	Marie Callender's	1/2 pie	2	3	10
pepperoni	Pappalo's Deep Dish	1/5 pie	2	2	5

PREPARED MEAL ITEM	SPECIFICATIONS	BRAND NAME	SERVING SIZE	PROTEIN BLOCKS	CARBOHYDRATE BLOCKS	FAT BLOCKS
Pizza, frozen (cont'd)	pepperoni	Pappalo's Deep Dish for One	1 pie	4	7	9
	pepperoni	Pappalo's for One	1 pie	4	5	9
	pepperoni	Pappalo's 9"	1/2 pie	3	4	6
	pepperoni	Pappalo's 12"	1/4 pie	3	4	6
	pepperoni	Tombstone Original 9"	1/3 pie	2	3	6
	pepperoni	Tombstone Original 12"	1/5 pie	2	3	6
	pepperoni	Tombstone for One	1 pie	4	4	12
	pepperoni	Tombstone for One 1/2 Less Fat	1 pie	4	5	4
	pepperoni	Tombstone Special Order 9"	1/3 pie	3	4	7
	pepperoni	Tombstone Special Order 12"	1/6 pie	2	3	6
	pepperoni	Totino's Microwave	1 pie	1	3	5
	pepperoni	Totino's Party	1/2 pie	2	3	7
	pepperoni	Totino's Party Family	1/3 pie	2	4	7
	pepperoni	Weight Watchers	1 pie	3	5	4
	pepperoni, double cheese	Tombstone Double Top	1/6 pie	3	3	7
	pepperoni, Italian	Tombstone Thin Crust	1/4 pie	3	3	9

sausage	Celeste for One	1 pie	3	5	9
sausage	Jeno's Crisp 'n Tasty	1 pie	2	5	9
sausage	Jeno's Microwave	1 pie	1	3	5
sausage	Pappalo's Deep Dish	1/5 pie	2	4	4
sausage	Pappalo's 9"	1/2 pie	3	5	6
sausage	Pappalo's 12"	1/4 pie	3	4	5
sausage	Tombstone Original 9"	1/3 pie	2	3	5
sausage	Tombstone Original 12"	1/5 pie	2	3	9
sausage	Totino's Microwave	1 pie	1	3	5
sausage	Totino's Party	1/2 pie	2	4	7
sausage	Totino's Party Family	1/4 pie	2	3	5
sausage, double cheese	Tombstone Double Top	1/6 pie	3	3	6
sausage, Italian	Tombstone For One	1 pie	4	4	11
sausage, Italian	Tombstone ThinCrust	1/4 pie	3	3	8
sausage, three	Tombstone Special Order 9"	1/3 pie	3	4	6
sausage, three	Tombstone Special Order 12"	1/6 pie	2	3	6
sausage/mushroom	Tombstone Original 12"	1/5 pie	2	3	5
sausage/pepperoni	Marie Callender's	1/2 pie	2	3	9

PREPARED MEAL ITEM	SPECIFICATIONS	BRAND NAME	SERVING SIZE	PROTEIN BLOCKS	CARBOHYDRATE BLOCKS	FAT BLOCKS
Pizza, frozen *(cont'd)*	sausage/pepperoni	Pappalo's Deep Dish	1/5 pie	2	4	5
	sausage/pepperoni	Pappalo's Deep Dish for One	1 pie	4	6	9
	sausage/pepperoni	Pappalo's for One	1 pie	4	5	9
	sausage/pepperoni	Pappalo's 9"	1/2 pie	3	5	6
	sausage/pepperoni	Pappalo's 12"	1/4 pie	3	4	6
	sausage/pepperoni	Tombstone Original 9"	1/3 pie	2	3	7
	sausage/pepperoni	Tombstone Original 12"	1/5 pie	2	3	6
	sausage/pepperoni	Tombstone For One	1 pie	4	4	12
	sausage/pepperoni	Totino's Select	1/3 pie	2	3	6
	sausage/pepperoni, double cheese	Tombstone Double Top	1/6 pie	3	3	7
	supreme	Jeno's Crisp 'n Tasty	1 pie	2	5	9
	supreme	Pappalo's Deep Dish	1/5 pie	3	4	5
	supreme	Pappalo's Deep Dish for One	1 pie	4	6	9
	supreme	Pappalo's for One	1 pie	4	5	9

supreme	Pappalo's 9"	1/3 pie	2	3	4
supreme	Pappalo's 12"	1/4 pie	3	4	5
supreme	Tombstone Original 12"	1/5 pie	2	3	6
supreme	Tombstone Light	1/5 pie	4	3	3
supreme, Italian	Tombstone ThinCrust	1/4 pie	3	3	8
supreme	Tombstone For One	1 pie	3	4	11
supreme	Tombstone For One 1/2 Less Fat	1 pie	4	5	4
supreme	Totino's Microwave	1 pie	1	3	6
supreme	Totino's Party	1/2 pie	2	4	7
supreme	Totino's Select	1/3 pie	2	3	6
supreme, super	Tombstone Special Order 9"	1/3 pie	3	4	7
supreme, super	Tombstone Special Order 12"	1/6 pie	2	3	6
tomato and mozzarella	Marie Callender's	1/2 pie	2	4	5
vegetable	Celeste for One	1 pie	3	5	8
vegetable	Tombstone Light	1/5 pie	4	3	2
vegetable	Tombstone For One 1/2 Less Fat	1 pie	4	5	3
vegetable, primavera	Marie Callender's	1/2 pie	2	4	5
	Empire Kosher	2-oz. pc.	1	2	2

Pizza, bagel

PREPARED MEAL ITEM	SPECIFICATIONS	BRAND NAME	SERVING SIZE	PROTEIN BLOCKS	CARBOHYDRATE BLOCKS	FAT BLOCKS
Pizza, croissant, frozen	cheese	Pepperidge Farm	1 pc.	2	4	7
	deluxe	Pepperidge Farm	1 pc.	2	4	9
	pepperoni	Pepperidge Farm	1 pc.	2	4	8
Pizza, English muffin		Empire Kosher	2-oz. pc.	1	2	2
Pizza, French bread, frozen	bacon cheddar	Stouffer's	1 pc.	2	4	7
	cheese	Healthy Choice	1 pc.	3	5	1
	cheese	Lean Cuisine	6 oz.	3	5	3
	cheese	Stouffer's	1 pc.	2	4	5
	cheese, double	Stouffer's	1 pc.	3	4	6
	cheeseburger	Stouffer's	1 pc.	3	3	9
	deluxe	Lean Cuisine	6 oz.	3	4	2
	deluxe	Stouffer's	1 pc.	3	4	7
	pepperoni	Healthy Choice	1 pc.	3	5	3
	pepperoni	Lean Cuisine	5 1/4 oz.	3	5	2
	pepperoni	Stouffer's	1 pc.	3	4	7

Pizza, Italian bread, frozen					
pepperoni and mushroom	Stouffer's	1 pc.	2	4	7
sausage	Healthy Choice	5 1/4 pc.	3	5	1
sausage	Stouffer's	1 pc.	3	4	7
sausage and pepperoni	Stouffer's	1 pc.	3	5	8
supreme	Healthy Choice	1 pc.	3	5	2
vegetable deluxe	Stouffer's	1 pc.	3	4	6
white	Stouffer's	1 pc.	2	4	9
cheese, four	Celeste	1 pc.	2	3	4
chicken, zesty	Celeste	1 pc.	2	3	3
deluxe	Celeste	1 pc.	2	4	4
pepperoni	Celeste	1 pc.	2	4	4
Pizza nuggets					
frozen	Hormel Quick Meal	5 pcs.	1	3	3
Pizza pocket, frozen	Amy's	1 pc.	2	4	3
deluxe	Lean Pockets	1 pc.	2	4	3
pepperoni	Croissant Pockets	1 pc.	2	4	5
pepperoni	Hot Pockets	1 pc.	2	4	6
pepperoni and sausage	Hot Pockets	1 pc.	2	4	5

PREPARED MEAL ITEM	SPECIFICATIONS	BRAND NAME	SERVING SIZE	PROTEIN BLOCKS	CARBOHYDRATE BLOCKS	FAT BLOCKS
Pizza pocket, frozen	sausage	Hot Pockets	1 pc.	2	4	5
(cont'd)	vegetable	Ken & Robert's Veggie Pockets	1 pc.	1	4	3
	vegetable, pepperoni style	Amy's	1 pc.	2	3	2
Pizza Pops	pepperoni	Totino's	1 pc.	2	3	5
	sausage, Italian	Totino's	1 pc.	2	3	5
	sausage/pepperoni	Totino's	1 pc.	2	3	6
	supreme	Totino's	1 pc.	2	3	5
Pizza rolls, frozen	cheese, three	Totino's	1 pc.	2	4	5
	combination	Totino's	1 pc.	2	4	6
	hamburger and cheese	Totino's	1 pc.	2	4	5
	meat, three	Totino's	1 pc.	2	4	5
	nacho and beef	Totino's	1 pc.	2	4	5
	pepperoni and cheese	Totino's	1 pc.	2	4	6
	sausage and cheese	Totino's	1 pc.	2	4	5
	sausage and mushroom	Totino's	1 pc.	2	4	5
	spicy, Italian style	Totino's	1 pc.	2	4	6

Pork dinner	frozen, barbeque	Swanson Hungry Man	1 pkg.	8	8	8	13
Pork entree, canned	chow mein	La Choy Bi-Pack	1 cup	1	1	1	1
Pork entree, freeze-dried	sweet and sour, w/rice	Mountain House	1 cup	1	1	4	3
Pork entree, frozen	cutlet	Banquet	1 pc.	2	2	4	8
	ribs, barbeque sauce	Swanson Fun Feast	1 pie	5	5	5	8
	rib-shape patty, barbeque	Swanson	1 pie	5	5	5	7
	sweet and sour	Chun King	1 pie	2	2	9	2
Pork sandwich	frozen, barbequed	Hormel Quick Meal	1 pc.	2	2	4	5
Potato dishes, canned	au gratin and bacon	Hormel	7 1/2 oz.	1	1	2	5
	scalloped, and ham	Hormel	7 1/2 oz.	1	1	2	5
	scalloped, and ham	Nalley's	7 1/2 oz.	1	1	3	2
	sliced, and beef	Dinty Moore	7 1/2 oz.	1	1	3	3
Potato dishes, frozen		Goya Rellenos de Papa	2 pcs.	2	2	3	3
		Goya Rellenos de Papa Cocktail	6 pcs.	1	1	3	3
	au gratin	Stouffer's Side Dish	4 1/2 oz.	1	1	2	2
	baked, butter flavor	Ore-Ida Twice Baked	5 oz.	1	1	2	3
	baked, cheddar	Ore-Ida Twice Baked	5 oz.	1	1	3	3

PREPARED MEAL ITEM	SPECIFICATIONS	BRAND NAME	SERVING SIZE	PROTEIN BLOCKS	CARBOHYDRATE BLOCKS	FAT BLOCKS
Potato dishes, frozen *(cont'd)*	baked, sour cream/chive	Ore-Ida Twice Baked	5 oz.	1	3	2
	baked, broccoli/cheese	The Budget Gourmet Light & Healthy	1 pkg.	2	4	3
	baked, broccoli/cheese	Ore-Ida Twice Baked	1 pkg.	1	3	1
	baked, broccoli/cheese	Weight Watchers	1 pkg.	2	3	2
	baked, broccoli/cheese, cheddar	Lean Cuisine Lunch Express	1 pkg.	2	3	2
	cheddar/cheddared	The Budget Gourmet Side Dish	5 oz.	1	2	3
	cheddar/cheddared	Lean Cuisine Deluxe	1 pkg.	2	3	2
	cheddar/cheddared, and broccoli	The Budget Gourmet Side Dish	5 oz.	1	2	3
	cheddar/cheddared, pocket scalloped	Ken & Robert's Veggie Pockets	1 pc.	1	4	3
	scalloped	Stouffer's Side Dish	5 oz.	1	2	2
	scalloped, and ham	Swanson	1 pkg.	3	3	4
	three cheese	The Budget Gourmet Side Dish	6 oz.	1	2	4

Radiatore entree	vegetarian, frozen	Hain Bolognese	10 oz.	2	5	1
Ravioli entree, canned	beef, tomato sauce	Franco-American	1 cup	1	4	2
	beef, tomato sauce	Hunt's Homestyle	1 cup	1	3	3
	beef, tomato sauce	Libby's	7 3/4 oz.	2	2	3
	beef, tomato sauce	Nalley's	1 cup	2	4	3
	beef, tomato sauce	Progresso	1 cup	1	5	2
	beef, tomato sauce	Top Shelf	10 oz.	3	3	3
	beef, tomato sauce	Chef Boyardee	1 cup	1	4	2
	beef, tomato sauce, w/meat	Franco-American	1 cup	2	4	3
	beef, tomato sauce, w/meat	Franco-American	1 cup	2	4	3
	beef, tomato sauce, mini, w/meat	Chef Boyardee Bowl	7 1/2 oz.	1	3	1
	cheese, tomato sauce	Chef Boyardee	1 cup	1	4	0
	cheese, tomato sauce	Progresso	1 cup	1	4	1

PREPARED MEAL ITEM	SPECIFICATIONS	BRAND NAME	SERVING SIZE	PROTEIN BLOCKS	CARBOHYDRATE BLOCKS	FAT BLOCKS
Ravioli entree, canned (cont'd)	cheese, tomato sauce, w/cheese	Chef Boyardee Bowl	7 1/2 oz.	1	4	0
	cheese, tomato sauce, w/meat	Chef Boyardee Bowl	7 1/2 oz.	1	3	1
	mini	Kid's Kitchen	7 1/2 oz.	1	4	2
	tomato sauce	Hormel Micro Cup	7 1/2 oz.	1	4	4
Ravioli entree, frozen, cheese		The Budget Gourmet Light & Healthy	1 pkg.	2	4	4
		Kid Cuisine Raptor	1 pkg.	1	6	2
		Swanson Fun Feast Roaring	1 pkg.	2	7	3
	cheese	Lean Cuisine	1 pkg.	2	3	2
	Florentine	Smart Ones	1 pkg.	1	4	1
	in marinara sauce	Marie Callender's	1 pkg.	2	5	5
	parmigiana	Healthy Choice	1 pkg.	2	4	1
Rice dishes, canned	Chinese fried	La Choy	1 cup	1	6	0
	Mexican	Old El Paso	1/2 cup	1	10	1

			P	C	F
Spanish	Old El Paso	1 cup	0	3	0
Spanish	Van de Kamp's	1 cup	0	4	1
Rice dishes, freeze-dried					
wild, pilaf, w/almonds	AlpineAire	1 1/3 cups	1	10	2
Rice dishes, frozen, see also Rice entree, frozen and specific listings					
Oriental w/vegetables	The Budget Gourmet	6 oz.	1	3	4
Rice dishes, mix					
pilaf, w/green beans	The Budget Gourmet	5 2/3 oz.	1	3	4
and beans, black	Carolina/Mahatma	2 oz. dry, approx. 1 cup prepared	1	4	1
and beans, black	Goya	2 oz. dry, approx. 1 cup prepared	1	3	0
and beans, black, mediterranean, pilaf	Near East	2 oz. dry, approx. 1 cup prepared	1	5	2
and beans, black, savory	Good Harvest	1/3 cup	1	3	1
and beans, black, spicy	Spice Island Quick	1 pkg.	1	3	0
and beans, Cajun	Lipton Rice & Sauce	1/2 pkg.	1	5	0

PREPARED MEAL ITEM	SPECIFICATIONS	BRAND NAME	SERVING SIZE	PROTEIN BLOCKS	CARBOHYDRATE BLOCKS	FAT BLOCKS
Rice dishes, mix (cont'd)	and beans, Cajun	Rice-A-Roni	1 cup, prepared	1	5	2
	and beans, pinto	Mahatma	2 oz. dry, approx.	1	4	0
			1 cup prepared			
	and beans, red	Carolina/Mahatma	2 oz. dry, approx.	1	4	0
			1 cup prepared			
	and beans, red	Goya	2 oz. dry, approx.	1	4	0
			1 cup prepared			
	and beans, red	Rice-A-Roni	1 cup, prepared	1	5	2
	and beans, red, pilaf	Near East	2 oz. dry, approx.	1	4	1
			1 cup prepared			
	and beans, red, spicy	Good Harvest	1/3 cup	1	3	0
	and beans, red, spicy	Spice Island Quick Meal	1 pkg.	1	3	1
	and beans, Spanish	Fantastic Only A Pinch Cup	2.2 oz.	1	5	1
	and beans, tomato	Near East	2 oz. dry, approx.	1	5	2
	herb, pilaf		1 cup prepared			

and beans, vegetables, garden, pilaf	Near East	2 oz. dry, approx. 1 cup prepared	1	5	2
beef/beef flavor	Country Inn	2 oz. dry, approx. 1 cup prepared	1	5	1
beef/beef flavor	Golden Saute	1/3 pkg.	1	5	1
beef/beef flavor	Lipton Rice & Sauce	1/2 pkg.	1	5	0
beef/beef flavor	Rice-A-Roni	1 cup, prepared	1	5	3
beef/beef flavor	Rice-A-Roni Less Salt	1 cup, prepared	1	6	2
beef/beef flavor	Success	2 oz. dry, approx. 1 cup prepared	1	5	0
beef/beef flavor, broccoli	Lipton Rice & Sauce	1/2 pkg.	1	5	0
beef/beef flavor, and mushroom	Rice-A-Roni	1 cup, prepared	1	5	2
beef/beef flavor, pilaf	Near East	2 oz. dry, approx. 1 cup prepared	1	5	2
broccoli, Alfredo	Lipton Rice & Sauce	1/2 pkg.	1	5	2

PREPARED MEAL ITEM	SPECIFICATIONS	BRAND NAME	SERVING SIZE	PROTEIN BLOCKS	CARBOHYDRATE BLOCKS	FAT BLOCKS
Rice dishes, mix *(cont'd)*	broccoli, cheese	Mahatma	2 oz. dry, approx. 1 cup prepared	1	4	1
	broccoli, cheese	Rice-A-Roni Fast	1 cup, prepared	1	4	4
	broccoli, cheese	Success	2 oz. dry, approx. 1 cup prepared	1	4	2
	broccoli au gratin	Country Inn	2 oz. dry, approx. 1 cup prepared	1	4	1
	broccoli au gratin	Rice-A-Roni	1 cup, prepared	1	5	6
	broccoli au gratin	Rice-A-Roni Less Salt	1 cup, prepared	1	5	4
	broccoli au gratin	Savory Classics	1 cup, prepared	1	5	2
	brown and wild	Success	2 oz. dry, approx. 1 cup prepared	1	4	0
	brown and wild, herb	Arrowhead Quick	1/4 pkg.	1	3	0
	Cajun	Lipton Rice & Sauce	2 oz. dry, approx. 1 cup prepared	1	5	0

cheddar, white, w/herbs	Rice-A-Roni	1 cup, prepared	1	5	5
cheddar, broccoli	Lipton Rice & Sauce	1/2 pkg.	1	5	1
cheese	Country Inn	2 oz. dry, approx. 1 cup prepared	1	4	1
chicken/chicken flavor	Country Inn	2 oz. dry, approx. 1 cup prepared	1	5	0
chicken/chicken flavor	Golden Saute	1/3 pkg.	1	5	2
chicken/chicken flavor	Lipton Rice & Sauce	1/2 pkg.	1	5	1
chicken/chicken flavor	Rice-A-Roni	1 cup, prepared	1	6	3
chicken/chicken flavor	Rice-A-Roni Less Salt	1 cup, prepared	1	6	2
chicken/chicken flavor	Rice-A-Roni Fast	1 cup, prepared	1	4	2
chicken/chicken flavor	Savory Classics	1 cup, prepared	1	6	3
chicken/chicken flavor	Success Classic	2 oz. dry, approx. 1 cup prepared	1	3	0
chicken/chicken flavor, creamy	Lipton Rice & Sauce	1/2 pkg.	1	5	2
chicken/chicken flavor, pilaf	Eastern Traditions	2 oz. dry, approx. 1 cup prepared	1	4	0

PREPARED MEAL ITEM	SPECIFICATIONS	BRAND NAME	SERVING SIZE	PROTEIN BLOCKS	CARBOHYDRATE BLOCKS	FAT BLOCKS
Rice dishes, mix (cont'd)	chicken/chicken flavor, pilaf	Knorr	1/3 cup	1	5	0
	chicken/chicken flavor, pilaf	Lundberg Quick Country	2 oz. dry, approx. 1 cup prepared	1	5	1
	chicken/chicken flavor, pilaf	Spice Island Quick	1 pkg.	1	4	0
	chicken/chicken flavor, pilaf, w/wild rice, Mediterranean	Near East	2 oz. dry, approx. 1 cup prepared	1	5	1
	chicken and broccoli	Country Inn	2 oz. dry, approx. 1 cup prepared	1	5	1
	chicken and broccoli	Golden Saute	1/2 pkg.	1	5	2
	chicken and broccoli	Lipton Rice & Sauce	1/2 pkg.	1	5	1
	chicken and broccoli	Rice-A-Roni	1 cup, prepared	1	5	2
	chicken and mushrooms	Rice-A-Roni	1 cup, prepared	1	6	5
	chicken w/vegetables	Country Inn	2 oz. dry, approx. 1 cup prepared	1	5	1

chicken w/vegetables	Rice-A-Roni	1 cup, prepared	1	6	2
chicken and wild rice	Country Inn	2 oz. dry, approx.	1	4	0
		1 cup prepared			
chicken and wild rice, almond	Savory Classics	1 cup, prepared	1	6	3
chili	Lundberg One Step	2 oz. dry, approx.	1	4	0
		1 cup prepared			
curry	Lundberg One Step	2 oz. dry, approx.	1	4	1
		1 cup prepared			
curry, pilaf	Near East	2 oz. dry, approx.	1	5	1
		1 cup prepared			
fried	Golden Saute	1/2 pkg.	1	5	0
fried	Rice-A-Roni	1 cup, prepared	1	6	4
garlic basil	Lundberg One Step	2 oz. dry, approx.	1	4	0
		1 cup prepared			
gumbo	Mahatma	2 oz. dry, approx.	0	3	1
		1 cup prepared			
herb, savory	Golden Saute	1/3 pkg.	1	5	2

PREPARED MEAL ITEM	SPECIFICATIONS	BRAND NAME	SERVING SIZE	PROTEIN BLOCKS	CARBOHYDRATE BLOCKS	FAT BLOCKS
Rice dishes, mix (cont'd)	herb and butter	Golden Saute	1/3 pkg.	1	5	2
	herb and butter	Lipton Rice & Sauce	1/2 pkg.	1	5	1
	herb and butter	Rice-A-Roni	1 cup, prepared	1	6	3
	jambalaya	Mahatma	2 oz. dry, approx. 1 cup prepared	1	5	0
	long grain and wild	Lipton Rice & Sauce Original	1/2 pkg.	1	5	0
	long grain and wild	Mahatma	2 oz. dry, approx. 1 cup prepared	1	4	0
	long grain and wild	Rice-A-Roni	1 cup, prepared	1	5	2
	long grain and wild	Uncle Ben's Fast	2 oz. dry, approx. 1 cup prepared	1	4	0
	long grain and wild	Uncle Ben's Original	2 oz. dry, approx. 1 cup prepared	1	4	0
	long grain and wild, butter and herb	Uncle Ben's	2 oz. dry, approx. 1 cup prepared	1	4	1

long grain and wild, chicken w/almonds	Rice-A-Roni	1 cup, prepared	1	5	3
long grain and wild, chicken and herbs	Uncle Ben's	2 oz. dry, approx. 1 cup prepared	1	4	1
long grain and wild, mushroom and herb	Lipton Rice & Sauce	1/2 pkg.	1	5	1
long grain and wild, pilaf	Near East	2 oz. dry, approx. 1 cup prepared	1	4	2
long grain and wild, pilaf	Rice-A-Roni	1 cup, prepared	1	5	2
long grain and wild, vegetable herb	Uncle Ben's	2 oz. dry, approx. 1 cup prepared	1	4	1
medley	Lipton Rice & Sauce	1/2 pkg.	1	5	1
Mexican	Goya	2 oz. dry, approx. 1 cup prepared	0	4	0
Mexican	Pritikin	2 oz. dry, approx. 1 cup prepared	1	4	1
Mexican	Savory Classics Fiesta	1 cup, prepared	1	6	2
mushroom	Lipton Rice & Sauce	1/2 pkg.	1	5	0

PREPARED MEAL ITEM	SPECIFICATIONS	BRAND NAME	SERVING SIZE	PROTEIN BLOCKS	CARBOHYDRATE BLOCKS	FAT BLOCKS
Rice dishes, mix (cont'd)	mushroom, brown	Uncle Ben's	2 oz. dry, approx.	1	4	1
			1 cup prepared			
	onion mushroom	Golden Saute	1/3 pkg.	1	5	1
	Oriental	Golden Saute	1/3 pkg.	1	5	2
	Oriental	Lipton Rice & Sauce	1/2 pkg.	1	5	1
	Oriental	Pritikin	2 oz. dry, approx.	1	4	1
			1 cup prepared			
	Oriental	Rice-A-Roni	2 oz. dry, approx.	1	6	2
			1 cup prepared			
	Oriental	Rice-A-Roni Fast	1 cup, prepared	1	5	4
	Oriental	Savory Classics	1 cup, prepared	1	5	4
	Oriental, and vegetables	Spice Island Quick	1 pkg.	1	4	1
	pilaf, see also specific listings	Casbah	1 oz.	0	2	0
	pilaf	Country Inn	2 oz. dry, approx.	1	5	0
			1 cup prepared			

pilaf	Eastern Traditions	2 oz. dry, approx. 1 cup prepared	1	5	0
pilaf	Eastern Traditions Harvest	2 oz. dry, approx. 1 cup prepared	1	4	0
pilaf	Knorr Original	1/3 cup	1	5	0
pilaf	Lipton Rice & Sauce	1/2 pkg.	1	5	0
pilaf	Mahatma	2 oz. dry, approx. 1 cup prepared	1	5	0
pilaf	Near East	2 oz. dry, approx. 1 cup prepared	1	5	2
pilaf	Rice-A-Roni	1 cup, prepared	1	6	3
pilaf	Success	2 oz. dry, approx. 1 cup prepared	1	5	0
pilaf, almond, toasted	Near East	2 oz. dry, approx. 1 cup prepared	1	4	2
pilaf, brown rice	Near East	2 oz. dry, approx. 1 cup prepared	1	4	2

PREPARED MEAL ITEM	SPECIFICATIONS	BRAND NAME	SERVING SIZE	PROTEIN BLOCKS	CARBOHYDRATE BLOCKS	FAT BLOCKS
Rice dishes, mix (cont'd)	pilaf, brown rice, w/miso	Fantastic Foods	2 oz. dry, approx. 1 cup prepared	1	6	1
	pilaf, garden	Savory Classics	1 cup, prepared	1	4	2
	pilaf, garlic herb	Lundberg Quick	2 oz. dry, approx. 1 cup prepared	1	5	1
	pilaf, lemon herb, w/jasmine rice	Knorr Original	1/3 cup	1	6	1
	pilaf, Mediterranean	Good Harvest	1/3 cup	1	3	1
	pilaf, mushroom, savory	Lundberg Quick	2 oz. dry, approx. 1 cup prepared	1	4	1
	pilaf, nutted	Casbah	1 oz.	0	2	0
	pilaf, three grain	Fantastic Foods	2 oz. dry, approx. 1 cup prepared	1	5	1
	pilaf, primavera	Goya	2 oz. dry, approx. 1 cup prepared	1	4	0

Food	Brand	Serving	P	C	F
risotto	Rice-A-Roni	1 cup, prepared	1	5	3
risotto, broccoli au gratin	Knorr	1/3 cup	1	6	1
risotto, chicken	Lipton Rice & Sauce	1/2 pkg.	1	5	1
risotto, garlic primavera	Lundberg	1/4 cup	1	3	0
risotto, italian herb	Lundberg	1/4 cup	1	3	0
risotto, Milanese	Knorr	1/3 cup	1	7	0
risotto, mushroom	Knorr	1/3 cup	1	7	0
risotto, onion herb	Knorr	1/3 cup	1	7	0
risotto, Parmesan, creamy	Lundberg	1/4 cup	1	3	1
risotto, primavera	Knorr	1/3 cup	1	7	0
tomato basil	Lundberg	1/4 cup	1	3	0
tomato-wild mushroom	Good Harvest	1/3 cup	0	3	0
Spanish	Country Inn	2 oz. dry, approx. 1 cup prepared	1	5	0
Spanish	Golden Saute	1/2 pkg.	1	5	2
Spanish	Good Harvest	1/3 cup	1	3	0
Spanish	Lipton Rice & Sauce	1/2 pkg.	1	5	0

PREPARED MEAL ITEM	SPECIFICATIONS	BRAND NAME	SERVING SIZE	PROTEIN BLOCKS	CARBOHYDRATE BLOCKS	FAT BLOCKS
Rice dishes, mix *(cont'd)*	Spanish	Mahatma	2 oz. dry, approx. 1 cup prepared	1	4	0
	Spanish	Rice-A-Roni	1 cup, prepared	1	5	3
	Spanish	Success	2 oz. dry, approx. 1 cup prepared	1	5	0
	Spanish, brown	Arrowhead Mills Quick	1/4 cup.	1	3	0
	Spanish, brown rice pilaf	Fantastic Foods	2 oz. dry, approx. 1 cup prepared	1	6	1
	Spanish, pilaf	Casbah	1 oz.	0	2	0
	Spanish, pilaf	Knorr	1/3 cup	1	5	0
	Spanish, pilaf	Near East	2 oz. dry, approx. 1 cup prepared	1	5	2
	Spanish, pilaf, brown	Lundberg Quick Fiesta	2 oz. dry, approx. 1 cup prepared	1	4	1
	Stroganoff	Rice-A-Roni	1 cup, prepared	1	5	5
	vegetable, country	Spice Island Quick	1 pkg.	1	4	4

vegetable, herb	Arrowhead Mills	1/4 pkg.	1	3	0
wild and bean	Good Harvest	1/3 cup	1	3	1
wild and vegetables	Spice Islands Quick	1 pkg.	0	4	0
yellow	Goya	2 oz. dry, approx. 1 cup prepared	1	4	0
yellow, saffron	Carolina/Mahatma	2 oz. dry, approx. 1 cup prepared	1	5	0
and beans	Weight Watchers	1 pkg.	2	3	3
Rice entree, frozen, see also Rice dishes, frozen					
and broccoli	Green Giant	1 pkg.	1	1	4
and chicken, stir-fry	Lean Cuisine	1 pkg.	2	4	3
fried, w/chicken	Chun King	1 pkg.	1	4	2
fried, w/pork	Lean Cuisine	1 pkg.	2	5	2
Mexican, w/chicken	Weight Watchers	1 pkg.	1	4	3
pilaf Florentine	Weight Watchers	1 pkg.	1	5	2
risotto, w/cheese and mushrooms	Weight Watchers	1 pkg.	2	4	3

PREPARED MEAL ITEM	SPECIFICATIONS	BRAND NAME	SERVING SIZE	PROTEIN BLOCKS	CARBOHYDRATE BLOCKS	FAT BLOCKS
Rice entree, frozen, see also Rice dishes, frozen (cont'd)	and vegetables	Green Giant Medley	1 pkg.	1	1	1
	and vegetables, Hunan style	Weight Watchers	1 pkg.	1	3	2
	and vegetables, Oriental	Green Giant International	1 pkg.	1	4	0
	and vegetables, pilaf	Green Giant	1 pkg.	1	1	1
	and vegetables, white and wild	Green Giant	1 pkg.	1	1	2
	and vegetables, paella	Weight Watchers	1 pkg.	1	5	2
	and vegetables, Peking style	Weight Watchers	1 pkg.	1	5	2
Rigatoni, canned	Italian garden sauce	Hunt's Homestyle	1 cup	1	3	2
Rigatoni entree, frozen		Lean Cuisine	9 oz.	1	2	1
	cream sauce, w/broccoli, chicken	The Budget Gourmet Light & Healthy	11 oz.	2	0	2
	parmigiana	Marie Callender's	7 1/2 oz.	2	3	5
	parmigiana	Marie Callender's Multi Serve	8 oz.	2	1	11
Shells, pasta, stuffed, frozen, w/out sauce		Celentano	4 shells	2	3	5

			P	C	F
Shells, pasta, stuffed, entree					
broccoli	Celentano Value Pack	3 shells	2	2	4
Florentine	Celentano	1 pkg.	3	3	7
marinara	Celentano	1/2 of 14-oz. pkg.	2	2	5
	Celentano Great Choice	1 pkg.	2	4	1
	Celentano Value Pack	3 shells, 8 oz.	2	4	5
	Celentano Great Choice	1 pkg.	2	3	1
	Celentano	1 pkg.	2	3	2
	Healthy Choice	1 pkg.	4	6	1
frozen, Mariner	The Budget Gourmet Light & Healthy	11 oz.	2	4	2
Shrimp dinner					
Shrimp entree, canned					
chow mein	La Choy Bi-Pack	1 cup	0	1	0
Shrimp entree, frozen					
beer batter	Gorton's	6 pcs.	1	2	5
breaded	Gorton's	6 pcs.	1	2	4
breaded	Mrs. Paul's	1 pkg.	4	3	5
breaded	Van de Kamp's	7 pcs.	2	3	3
breaded, butterfly	Van de Kamp's	7 pcs.	2	3	5
breaded, w/pasta	Marie Callender's	1 cup	2	3	4

PREPARED MEAL ITEM	SPECIFICATIONS	BRAND NAME	SERVING SIZE	PROTEIN BLOCKS	CARBOHYDRATE BLOCKS	FAT BLOCKS
Shrimp entree, frozen	breaded, scampi	Gorton's	6 pcs.	1	2	5
(cont'd)	marinara	Healthy Choice	1 pkg.	1	4	0
	marinara	Smart Ones	1 pkg.	1	4	1
	popcorn, breaded	Gorton's	1 cup	1	2	5
	popcorn, breaded	Van de Kamp's	4 oz.	2	3	4
	popcorn, breaded, garlic and herb	Gorton's	3.5 oz.	2	3	4
	and vegetables	Healthy Choice	12.5 oz.	2	5	1
Sloppy Joe entree	frozen	Swanson Fun Feast	1 pkg.	2	4	3
Soup, canned, ready-to-serve	bean	Grandma Brown's	1 cup	1	2	1
	bean, black	Goya	1 cup	1	3	1
	bean, black	Progresso	1 cup	1	2	1
	bean, black, w/bacon	Old El Paso	1 cup	1	2	1
	bean, black and vegetables	Health Valley	1 cup	1	1	0

bean, salsa	Campbell's Home Cookin'	1 cup	0	3	0
bean w/bacon and ham	Campbell's Microwave	1 cup	1	2	2
bean and ham	Campbell's Chunky	1 cup	0	2	1
bean and ham	Campbell's Chunky	11 oz.	1	3	1
bean and ham	Campbell's Chunky Ham 'n Bean	11 oz.	2	3	3
bean and ham	Campbell's Home Cookin'	1 cup	0	3	1
bean and ham	Campbell's Home Cookin'	11 oz.	0	3	1
bean and ham	Healthy Choice	1 cup	1	3	1
bean and ham	Progresso	1 cup	1	2	1
beans and rice, creole	Campbell's Chunky	1 cup	1	2	3
beans and rice, creole	Campbell's Chunky	11 oz.	2	3	3
beef, barley	Progresso	1 cup	1	1	1
beef, barley	Progresso Hearty Classics	1 cup	1	2	1
beef, broth	Swanson	1 cup	0	0	0
beef, chunky	Campbell's Microwave	1 cup	1	2	2
beef, hearty	Old El Paso	1 cup	1	2	1
beef, minestrone	Progresso	1 cup	1	1	1
beef, noodle	Progresso	1 cup	1	2	1

PREPARED MEAL ITEM	SPECIFICATIONS	BRAND NAME	SERVING SIZE	PROTEIN BLOCKS	CARBOHYDRATE BLOCKS	FAT BLOCKS
Soup, canned,	beef, pasta	Campbell's Chunky	1 cup	1	2	1
ready-to-serve	beef, pasta	Campbell's Chunky	11 oz.	1	2	1
(cont'd)	beef, potato	Healthy Choice	1 cup	1	1	1
	beef Stroganoff	Campbell's Chunky	1 cup	3	3	5
	beef vegetable	Progresso Healthy Classics	1 cup	1	2	1
	beef vegetable, country	Campbell's Chunky	1 cup	1	2	1
	beef vegetable, country	Campbell's Chunky	11 oz.	1	2	2
	beef vegetable and rotini	Progresso Pasta Soup	1 cup	1	1	1
	borscht	Gold's	1 cup	0	2	0
	broccoli, carotene	Health Valley	1 cup	1	1	0
	broccoli, cream of	Progresso Healthy Classics	1 cup	0	1	1
	broccoli and shells	Progresso Pasta Soup	1 cup	0	1	0
	broccoli cheese	Campbell's Chunky	1 cup	2	1	4
	chicken	Campbell's Chunky Old Fashioned	1 cup	1	1	1
	chicken	Campbell's Chunky Old Fashioned	11 oz.	1	2	2

chicken	Progresso Chickarina	1 cup	1	1	2
chicken barley	Progresso	1 cup	1	1	1
chicken, hearty	Healthy Choice	1 cup	1	2	1
chicken, hearty	Progresso	11 oz.	1	1	1
chicken, minestrone	Progresso	1 cup	1	1	1
chicken, cream of	Campbell's Home Cookin'	1 cup	3	1	6
chicken, cream of	Campbell's Home Cookin'	11 oz.	3	1	7
chicken, cream of	Progresso	1 cup	1	1	3
chicken, cream of, w/mushrooms	Healthy Choice	1 cup	1	2	1
chicken, cream of, w/vegetables	Healthy Choice	1 cup	1	2	1
chicken broth	Campbell's Low Sodium	11 oz.	0	0	1
chicken broth	Campbell's Healthy Request	1 cup	0	0	0
chicken broth	College Inn	1 cup	0	0	1
chicken broth	College Inn Less Sodium	1 cup	0	0	1
chicken broth	Pritikin	1 cup	0	0	0
chicken broth	Progresso	1 cup	0	0	0

PREPARED MEAL ITEM	SPECIFICATIONS	BRAND NAME	SERVING SIZE	PROTEIN BLOCKS	CARBOHYDRATE BLOCKS	FAT BLOCKS
Soup, canned, ready-to-serve *(cont'd)*	chicken broth	Swanson	1 cup	0	0	1
	chicken broth	Swanson Natural Goodness	1 cup	0	0	0
	chicken chowder, corn	Campbell's Healthy Request	1 cup	1	2	1
	chicken chowder, mushroom	Campbell's Chunky	1 cup	2	1	4
	chicken noodle	Campbell's Chunky Classic	1 cup	1	2	1
	chicken noodle	Campbell's Chunky Classic	11 oz.	1	2	1
	chicken noodle	Campbell's Home Cookin'	1 cup	1	1	1
	chicken noodle	Campbell's Home Cookin'	11 oz.	1	1	1
	chicken noodle	Campbell's Low Sodium	11 oz.	1	2	2
	chicken noodle	Campbell's Microwave	1 container	1	1	1
	chicken noodle	Healthy Choice Old Fashioned	1 cup	1	2	1
	chicken noodle	Progresso	1 cup	1	1	1
	chicken noodle	Progresso	11 oz.	1	1	1
	chicken noodle	Progresso Healthy Classics	1 cup	1	1	1
	chicken noodle	Weight Watchers	11 oz.	1	2	1

Food	Brand	Serving	P	C	F
chicken noodle, chunky	Campbell's Microwave	1 container	1	2	2
chicken noodle, creamy	Campbell's Chunky	1 cup	3	1	6
chicken noodle, creamy	Campbell's Chunky	11 oz.	3	1	7
chicken noodle, hearty	Campbell's Healthy Request	1 cup	1	3	1
chicken noodle, hearty	Old El Paso	1 cup	1	1	1
chicken noodle, w/mushrooms	Campbell's Chunky	1 cup	1	1	1
chicken pasta	Healthy Choice	1 cup	1	2	1
chicken pasta	Pritikin	1 cup	1	2	0
chicken pasta, penne, spicy	Progresso Pasta Soup	1 cup	1	1	1
chicken rice	Campbell's Chunky	1 cup	1	2	1
chicken rice	Campbell's Home Cookin'	1 cup	0	2	1
chicken rice	Campbell's Home Cookin'	11 oz.	0	2	1
chicken rice	Campbell's Microwave	1 cup	0	2	1
chicken rice	Campbell's Healthy Request	1 cup	0	2	1
chicken rice	Old El Paso	1 cup	1	1	1
chicken rice	Pritikin	1 cup	1	1	0
chicken rice	Weight Watchers	11 oz.	1	1	1

PREPARED MEAL ITEM	SPECIFICATIONS	BRAND NAME	SERVING SIZE	PROTEIN BLOCKS	CARBOHYDRATE BLOCKS	FAT BLOCKS
Soup, canned, ready-to-serve (cont'd)	chicken rice, w/rice	Campbell's Microwave	1 cup	1	1	1
	chicken rice, w/rice	Healthy Choice	1 cup	1	2	1
	chicken rice, w/vegetables	Progresso	1 cup	1	1	1
	chicken rice, w/vegetables	Progresso	11 oz.	1	2	1
	chicken rice, w/vegetables	Progresso Healthy Classics	1 cup	1	1	1
	chicken rice, wild rice	Progresso	1 cup	1	1	1
	chicken rice and rotini	Progresso Pasta Soup	1 cup	1	1	1
	chicken vegetable	Campbell's Chunky	1 cup	0	1	0
	chicken vegetable	Campbell's Home Cookin'	1 cup	1	2	1
	chicken vegetable	Campbell's Home Cookin'	11 oz.	1	2	1
	chicken vegetable	Old El Paso	1 cup	1	1	1
	chicken vegetable	Progresso Homestyle	1 cup	1	1	1
	chicken vegetable, hearty	Campbell's Healthy Request	1 cup	0	2	1
	chicken vegetable, nuggets	Campbell's Chunky	1 cup	1	2	2
	chicken vegetable, nuggets	Campbell's Chunky	11 oz.	1	2	2
	chicken vegetable and penne	Progresso Pasta Soup	1 cup	1	1	1

chili beef w/beans	Campbell's Chunky	1 cup	1	3	2
chili beef w/beans	Campbell's Chunky	11 oz.	1	3	2
chili beef w/beans	Campbell's Microwave	1 container	1	2	2
chili beef w/beans	Healthy Choice	1 cup	1	3	0
clam chowder, Manhattan	Campbell's Chunky	1 cup	1	2	1
clam chowder, Manhattan	Campbell's Chunky	11 oz.	1	2	1
clam chowder, Manhattan	Progresso	1 cup	1	1	1
clam chowder, New England	Campbell's Chunky	1 cup	2	2	5
clam chowder, New England	Campbell's Chunky	11 oz.	3	3	6
clam chowder, New England	Campbell's Home Cookin'	1 cup	3	1	5
clam chowder, New England	Campbell's Microwave	1 container	2	1	5
clam chowder, New England	Campbell's Healthy Request	1 cup	1	2	1
clam chowder, New England	Healthy Choice	1 cup	1	2	0
clam chowder, New England	Progresso	1 cup	1	2	3
clam chowder, New England	Progresso	11 oz.	1	2	1
clam chowder, New England	Progresso Healthy Classics	1 cup	1	2	1
clam chowder, New England, chunky	Campbell's Microwave	1 container	3	3	6

PREPARED MEAL ITEM	SPECIFICATIONS	BRAND NAME	SERVING SIZE	PROTEIN BLOCKS	CARBOHYDRATE BLOCKS	FAT BLOCKS
Soup, canned, ready-to-serve (cont'd)	clam rotini chowder	Progresso Pasta Soup	1 cup	1	2	3
	corn, country, and vegetable	Health Valley	1 cup	1	1	0
	corn chowder	Campbell's Chunky	1 cup	2	2	5
	corn chowder	Campbell's Chunky	11 oz.	3	2	6
	corn chowder	Progresso	1 cup	1	2	3
	corn chowder, chicken	Healthy Choice	1 cup	1	3	1
	egg flower	Rice Road	1 cup	0	2	1
	escarole, in chicken broth	Progresso	1 cup	0	0	0
	garlic pasta	Progresso Healthy Classics	1 cup	0	2	1
	hot and sour	Rice Road	1 cup	0	1	1
	Italian, carotene	Health Valley Fat Free	1 cup	1	1	0
	lentil	Healthy Choice	1 cup	1	3	0
	lentil	Pritikin	1 cup	1	2	0
	lentil	Progresso	1 cup	1	2	1
	lentil	Progresso	11 oz.	1	2	1

lentil	Progresso Healthy Classics	1 cup	1	2	1
lentil and carrots	Health Valley Fat Free	1 cup	1	1	0
lentil, hearty	Campbell's Home Cookin'	1 cup	0	2	0
lentil, hearty	Campbell's Home Cookin'	11 oz.	1	3	1
lentil w/sausage	Progresso	1 cup	1	2	2
lentil and shells	Progresso Pasta Soup	1 cup	1	2	1
macaroni and bean	Progresso	1 cup	1	2	1
meatballs and pasta pearls	Progresso Pasta Soup	1 cup	1	1	2
minestrone	Campbell's Chunky	1 cup	1	2	2
minestrone	Healthy Choice	1 cup	1	2	0
minestrone	Pritikin	1 cup	1	2	0
minestrone	Progresso	1 cup	1	2	1
minestrone	Progresso	11 oz.	1	2	1
minestrone	Progresso Healthy Classics	1 cup	1	2	1
minestrone	Weight Watchers	11 oz.	1	2	1
minestrone, hearty	Campbell's Healthy Request	1 cup	0	2	1
minestrone, Italian	Health Valley	1 cup	1	1	0

PREPARED MEAL ITEM	SPECIFICATIONS	BRAND NAME	SERVING SIZE	PROTEIN BLOCKS	CARBOHYDRATE BLOCKS	FAT BLOCKS
Soup, canned, ready-to-serve (cont'd)	minestrone, shells	Progresso Pasta Soup	1 cup	1	2	1
	minestrone, Tuscany	Campbell's Home Cookin'	1 cup	1	2	2
	minestrone, Tuscany	Campbell's Home Cookin'	11 oz.	1	2	3
	minestrone, zesty	Progresso	1 cup	1	1	2
	mushroom, cream of	Campbell's Home Cookin'	1 cup	2	1	4
	mushroom, cream of	Campbell's Home Cookin'	1 cup	3	1	6
	mushroom, cream of	Campbell's Low Sodium	1 cup	2	2	5
	mushroom, cream of	Healthy Choice	1 cup	0	2	0
	mushroom, cream of	Progresso	1 cup	0	1	3
	mushroom rice	Campbell's Home Cookin'	1 cup	0	2	0
	Oriental broth	Swanson	1 cup	0	0	0
	pasta Bolognese	Health Valley Healthy Pasta	1 cup	1	1	0
	pasta, cacciatore	Health Valley Healthy Pasta	1 cup	1	2	0
	pasta, Chinese	Rice Road	1 cup	0	1	1
	pasta, fagioli	Health Valley Healthy Pasta	1 cup	1	1	0

primavera	Health Valley Healthy Pasta	1 cup	1	1	0
Romano	Health Valley Healthy Pasta	1 cup	1	2	0
pea, split	Campbell's Low Sodium	1 cup	1	4	1
pea, split	Grandma Brown's	1 cup	1	3	1
pea, split	Pritikin	1 cup	1	2	0
pea, split	Progresso Healthy Classics	1 cup	1	3	1
pea, split and carrots	Health Valley	1 cup	1	1	0
pea, split, green	Progresso	1 cup	1	2	1
pea, split, w/ham	Campbell's Chunky	1 cup	1	3	1
pea, split, w/ham	Campbell's Chunky	11 oz.	1	3	1
pea, split, w/ham	Campbell's Home Cookin'	1 cup	0	3	1
pea, split, w/ham	Campbell's Home Cookin'	11 oz.	0	3	1
pea, split, w/ham	Campbell's Healthy Request	1 cup	0	3	1
pea, split, w/ham	Healthy Choice	1 cup	1	3	1
pea, split, w/ham	Progresso	1 cup	1	2	1
penne, hearty, chicken broth	Progresso Pasta Soup	1 cup	1	1	0
penne, zesty	Campbell's Healthy Request	1 cup	0	2	0

PREPARED MEAL ITEM	SPECIFICATIONS	BRAND NAME	SERVING SIZE	PROTEIN BLOCKS	CARBOHYDRATE BLOCKS	FAT BLOCKS
Soup, canned,	pepper steak	Campbell's Chunky	1 cup	0	2	1
ready-to-serve	pepper steak	Campbell's Chunky	11 oz.	1	2	1
(cont'd)	potato ham chowder	Campbell's Chunky	11 oz.	3	2	6
	sirloin burger, chunky	Campbell's Microwave	1 cup	1	2	3
	sirloin burger, w/vegetable	Campbell's Chunky	1 cup	1	2	3
	steak and potato	Campbell's Chunky	1 cup	1	2	1
	steak and potato	Campbell's Chunky	11 oz.	1	2	2
	tomato	Campbell's Low Sodium	11 oz.	1	3	2
	tomato	Progresso	1 cup	0	1	1
	tomato, beef and rotini	Progresso	1 cup	1	1	2
	tomato, garden	Campbell's Home Cookin'	11 oz.	1	3	1
	tomato, garden	Healthy Choice	1 cup	1	2	1
	tomato, hearty, rotini	Progresso Pasta Soup	1 cup	0	1	0
	tomato, tortellini	Progresso Pasta Soup	1 cup	1	1	2
	tomato, vegetable	Campbell's Healthy Request	1 cup	0	2	1

tomato, vegetable	Health Valley	1 cup	1	1	0
tomato, vegetable, garden	Progresso Healthy Classics	1 cup	0	2	0
tortellini, in chicken broth	Progresso	1 cup	0	1	1
tortellini, creamy	Progresso	1 cup	1	2	5
turkey w/wild rice	Healthy Choice	1 cup	1	1	1
turkey w/wild rice, vegetable	Campbell's Healthy Request	1 cup	0	2	1
vegetable	Campbell's Chunky	1 cup	1	2	1
vegetable	Campbell's Chunky	11 oz.	1	3	1
vegetable	Campbell's Microwave	1 container	0	2	1
vegetable	Campbell's Healthy Request	1 cup	0	2	0
vegetable	Progresso	1 cup	0	1	1
vegetable	Progresso Healthy Classics	1 cup	0	1	1
vegetable	Weight Watchers	11 oz.	0	2	1
vegetable, barley	Health Valley Fat Free	1 cup	1	2	0
vegetable, carotene	Health Valley Fat Free	1 cup	1	1	0
vegetable, country	Campbell's Home Cookin'	1 cup	0	2	0

PREPARED MEAL ITEM	SPECIFICATIONS	BRAND NAME	SERVING SIZE	PROTEIN BLOCKS	CARBOHYDRATE BLOCKS	FAT BLOCKS
Soup, canned, ready-to-serve (cont'd)	vegetable, country	Campbell's Home Cookin'	11 oz.	0	3	1
	vegetable, country	Healthy Choice	1 cup	0	2	0
	vegetable, 5 bean	Health Valley	1 cup	1	2	0
	vegetable, 14 garden	Health Valley Fat Free	1 cup	1	1	0
	vegetable, garden	Healthy Choice	1 cup	1	3	0
	vegetable, garden	Old El Paso	1 cup	1	2	1
	vegetable, harborside	Campbell's Home Cookin'	1 cup	0	1	1
	vegetable, hearty	Campbell's Healthy Request	1 cup	0	2	0
	vegetable, hearty	Pritikin	1 cup	0	2	0
	vegetable, hearty, w/pasta	Campbell's Chunky	1 cup	1	2	1
	vegetable, hearty, w/rotini	Progresso Pasta Soup	1 cup	0	2	0
	vegetable, Italian	Campbell's Home Cookin'	1 cup	1	1	1
	vegetable, Italian	Campbell's Home Cookin'	11 oz.	1	2	2
	vegetable, Mediterranean	Campbell's Chunky	1 cup	1	2	2
	vegetable, Southwestern	Campbell's Home Cookin'	1 cup	0	2	1

vegetable, Southwestern	Campbell's Healthy Request	1 cup	0	3	0
vegetable, vegetarian	Pritikin	1 cup	0	2	0
vegetable beef	Campbell's Chunky	1 cup	1	2	2
vegetable beef	Campbell's Chunky	11 oz.	1	2	2
vegetable beef	Campbell's Home Cookin'	1 cup	0	2	1
vegetable beef	Campbell's Home Cookin'	11 oz.	0	2	1
vegetable beef	Campbell's Low Sodium	11 oz.	1	2	2
vegetable beef	Campbell's Microwave	1 container	0	1	1
vegetable beef	Healthy Choice	1 cup	1	2	0
vegetable beef, hearty	Campbell's Healthy Request	1 cup	0	2	1
vegetable broth	Pritikin	1 cup	0	0	0
vegetable broth	Swanson	1 cup	0	0	0
Soup, canned, condensed					
asparagus, cream of	Campbell's	1/2 cup	1	1	2
bean, w/bacon	Campbell's	1/2 cup	1	2	2
bean, w/bacon	Campbell's Healthy Request	1/2 cup	0	2	1
bean, black	Campbell's	1/2 cup	0	2	1

PREPARED MEAL ITEM	SPECIFICATIONS	BRAND NAME	SERVING SIZE	PROTEIN BLOCKS	CARBOHYDRATE BLOCKS	FAT BLOCKS
Soup, canned, condensed *(cont'd)*	beef, broth, double rich	Campbell's	1/2 cup	0	0	0
	beef, consomme	Campbell's	1/2 cup	0	0	0
	beef, noodle	Campbell's	1/2 cup	0	1	1
	beef, w/vegetables, barley	Campbell's	1/2 cup	0	1	1
	broccoli, cream of	Campbell's	1/2 cup	1	1	2
	broccoli, cream of	Campbell's Healthy Request	1/2 cup	0	1	1
	broccoli, cheese	Campbell's	1/2 cup	1	1	3
	celery, cream of	Campbell's	1/2 cup	1	1	2
	celery, cream of	Campbell's Reduced Fat	1/2 cup	1	1	1
	celery, cream of	Campbell's Healthy Request	1/2 cup	0	1	1
	cheese, cheddar	Campbell's	1/2 cup	1	1	3
	cheese, nacho	Campbell's	1/2 cup	1	1	3
	chicken, alphabet, w/vegetables	Campbell's	1/2 cup	0	1	1

chicken broth	Campbell's	1/2 cup	0	0	1
chicken, cream of	Campbell's	1/2 cup	1	1	3
chicken, cream of	Campbell's Reduced Fat	1/2 cup	1	1	1
chicken, cream of	Campbell's Healthy Request	1/2 cup	0	1	1
chicken, cream of, and broccoli	Campbell's	1/2 cup	1	1	3
chicken, cream of, and broccoli	Campbell's Healthy Request	1/2 cup	0	1	1
chicken, dumplings	Campbell's	1/2 cup	1	1	1
chicken, gumbo	Campbell's	1/2 cup	0	1	1
chicken mushroom, creamy	Campbell's	1/2 cup	1	1	3
chicken noodle	Campbell's	1/2 cup	0	1	1
chicken noodle	Campbell's Healthy Request	1/2 cup	0	1	1
chicken noodle, creamy	Campbell's	1/2 cup	1	1	2
chicken noodle	Campbell's Homestyle	1/2 cup	0	1	1
chicken noodle O's	Campbell's	1/2 cup	1	1	1

PREPARED MEAL ITEM	SPECIFICATIONS	BRAND NAME	SERVING SIZE	PROTEIN BLOCKS	CARBOHYDRATE BLOCKS	FAT BLOCKS
Soup, canned, condensed (cont'd)	chicken w/rice	Campbell's	1/2 cup	0	1	1
	chicken w/rice	Campbell's Healthy Request	1/2 cup	0	1	1
	chicken and stars	Campbell's	1/2 cup	0	1	1
	chicken, vegetable	Campbell's	1/2 cup	0	1	1
	chicken, vegetable	Campbell's Healthy Request	1/2 cup	0	1	1
	chicken, vegetable, Southwestern	Campbell's	1/2 cup	0	2	1
	chicken, wild rice	Campbell's	1/2 cup	0	1	1
	chicken wonton	Campbell's	1/2 cup	0	0	0
	chili beef w/beans	Campbell's	1/2 cup	1	2	2
	clam chowder, Manhattan	Campbell's	1/2 cup	0	1	0
	clam chowder, New England	Campbell's	1/2 cup	0	2	1
	clam chowder, New England	Doxsee	1/2 cup	0	2	1
	corn, golden	Campbell's	1/2 cup	1	2	1
	minestrone	Campbell's	1/2 cup	0	1	1

minestrone	Campbell's Healthy Request	1/2 cup	0	2	0
mushroom, beefy	Campbell's	1/2 cup	1	0	1
mushroom, cream of	Campbell's	1/2 cup	1	1	2
mushroom, cream of	Campbell's Reduced Fat	1/2 cup	1	1	1
mushroom, cream of	Campbell's Healthy Request	1/2 cup	0	1	1
mushroom, golden	Campbell's	1/2 cup	1	1	1
noodle, curly, chicken broth	Campbell's	1/2 cup	0	1	1.
noodle, double, chicken broth	Campbell's	1/2 cup	0	1	1
noodle and ground beef	Campbell's	1/2 cup	1	1	1
onion, creamy	Campbell's	1/2 cup	1	1	2
onion, French, w/beef stock	Campbell's	1/2 cup	0	1	1
oyster stew	Campbell's	1/2 cup	1	1	2
pea, green	Campbell's	1/2 cup	1	3	1
pea, split, w/ham and bacon	Campbell's	1/2 cup	1	3	1
pepper, cream of, Mexican	Campbell's	1/2 cup	1	1	2
pepperpot	Campbell's	1/2 cup	1	1	2
potato, cream of	Campbell's	1/2 cup	1	1	1

PREPARED MEAL ITEM	SPECIFICATIONS	BRAND NAME	SERVING SIZE	PROTEIN BLOCKS	CARBOHYDRATE BLOCKS	FAT BLOCKS
Soup, canned, condensed (cont'd)	Scotch broth	Campbell's	1/2 cup	1	1	1
	shrimp, cream of	Campbell's	1/2 cup	1	1	2
	tomato	Campbell's	1/2 cup	0	2	1
	tomato	Campbell's Healthy Request	1/2 cup	0	2	1
	tomato, bisque	Campbell's	1/2 cup	1	2	1
	tomato, cream of	Campbell's Homestyle	1/2 cup	0	2	1
	tomato, fiesta	Campbell's	1/2 cup	0	2	0
	tomato, italian, w/basil, oregano	Campbell's	1/2 cup	0	2	0
	tomato, rice	Campbell's Old Fashioned	1/2 cup	0	2	1
	turkey noodle	Campbell's	1/2 cup	0	1	1
	turkey, vegetable	Campbell's	1/2 cup	0	1	1
	vegetable	Campbell's	1/2 cup	0	1	1
	vegetable	Campbell's Homestyle	1/2 cup	0	1	1
	vegetable	Campbell's Old Fashioned	1/2 cup	0	1	1

			Protein	Carbohydrate	Fat
vegetable	Campbell's Healthy Request	1/2 cup	0	2	0
vegetable beef	Campbell's	1/2 cup	0	1	1
vegetable beef	Campbell's Healthy Request	1/2 cup	0	1	1
vegetable, California style	Campbell's	1/2 cup	0	1	0
vegetable, hearty	Campbell's Healthy Request	1/2 cup	0	2	0
vegetable, hearty, w/pasta	Campbell's	1/2 cup	0	2	0
vegetable, vegetarian	Campbell's	1/2 cup	0	1	0
bacon, lettuce, tomato w/chicken broth	Pepperidge Farm	3/4 cup	1	1	2
Soup, canned, semi-condensed, undiluted					
black bean w/sherry	Pepperidge Farm	3/4 cup	0	2	1
broccoli, cream of	Pepperidge Farm	3/4 cup	1	1	2
chicken curry	Pepperidge Farm	3/4 cup	1	2	3
chicken w/rice	Pepperidge Farm	3/4 cup	1	1	1
chicken w/rice, w/bacon and ham	Campbell's	3/4 cup	1	2	1
clam chowder, Manhattan	Pepperidge Farm	3/4 cup	0	1	1

PREPARED MEAL ITEM	SPECIFICATIONS	BRAND NAME	SERVING SIZE	PROTEIN BLOCKS	CARBOHYDRATE BLOCKS	FAT BLOCKS
Soup, canned,	clam chowder, New England	Pepperidge Farm	3/4 cup	1	1	3
semi-condensed,	consomme, Madrilene	Pepperidge Farm	3/4 cup	0	1	0
undiluted (cont'd)	corn chowder	Pepperidge Farm	3/4 cup	1	1	3
	crab	Pepperidge Farm	3/4 cup	0	1	1
	gazpacho	Pepperidge Farm	3/4 cup	0	1	1
	hunter's, w/turkey, beef	Pepperidge Farm	3/4 cup	1	1	2
	lobster bisque	Pepperidge Farm	3/4 cup	2	1	4
	minestrone	Pepperidge Farm	3/4 cup	1	1	1
	mushroom, shiitake	Pepperidge Farm	3/4 cup	1	1	1
	onion, French	Pepperidge Farm	3/4 cup	0	1	0
	oyster stew	Pepperidge Farm	3/4 cup	2	1	3
	pea, green, w/ham	Pepperidge Farm	3/4 cup	1	3	2
	vichyssoise	Pepperidge Farm	3/4 cup	1	1	3
	watercress	Pepperidge Farm	3/4 cup	1	1	1
Soup, frozen	barley mushroom	Tabatchnik	1 cup	0	1	0

			Protein	Carbohydrate	Fat
barley mushroom, no salt	Tabatchnik	1 cup	0	1	0
bean, Yankee	Tabatchnik	1 cup	1	2	1
broccoli, cream of	Tabatchnik	1 cup	0	1	1
cabbage	Tabatchnik	1 cup	0	1	0
cheddar vegetable, Wisconsin	Tabatchnik	1 cup	0	1	3
chicken w/noodles and dumplings	Tabatchnik	1 cup	0	1	1
chicken w/noodles and vegetables	Tabatchnik	1 cup	0	1	0
corn chowder	Tabatchnik	1 cup	0	2	2
lentil, Tuscany	Tabatchnik	1 cup	1	2	0
minestrone	Tabatchnik	1 cup	1	2	0
pea	Tabatchnik	1 cup	1	2	1
pea, no salt	Tabatchnik	1 cup	1	2	1
potato, New England	Tabatchnik	1 cup	0	2	2
potato, old-fashioned	Tabatchnik	1 cup	0	2	0

PREPARED MEAL ITEM	SPECIFICATIONS	BRAND NAME	SERVING SIZE	PROTEIN BLOCKS	CARBOHYDRATE BLOCKS	FAT BLOCKS
Soup, frozen (cont'd)	spinach, cream of	Tabatchnik	1 cup	0	1	1
	vegetable	Tabatchnik	1 cup	1	2	0
	vegetable, no salt	Tabatchnik	1 cup	1	2	0
	barley, vegetable, hearty	Fantastic Cup	1 pkg.	1	3	0
	bean	Bean Cuisine Bouillabaisse	1 serving	1	1	0
	bean, black	Bean Cuisine Island	1 serving	1	2	0
	bean, black	Knorr Cup	1 pkg.	1	3	0
	bean, black	Smart Soup	1 pkg.	1	2	1
	bean, black, hearty	Fantastic Jumpin' Cup	1 pkg.	1	3	0
	bean, black, Santa Fe	Campbell's Soupsations	1 pkg.	0	5	1
	bean, black, spicy, w/couscous	Health Valley	1/3 cup	1	3	0
	bean, black, zesty, w/rice	Health Valley	1/3 cup	1	2	0
	bean, 5, hearty	Fantastic Cup	1 pkg.	1	4	0
	bean, navy	Knorr Cup	1 pkg.	1	2	0
	bean, white	Bean Cuisine Provencale	1 serving	1	1	0

bean and ham	Hormel Micro Cup	1 pkg.	1	2	1
beef vegetable	Hormel Micro Cup	1 pkg.	1	1	0
broccoli-cheese, cheddar, creamy	Fantastic Cup	1 pkg.	1	2	1
broccoli-cheese, creamy	Cup-a-Soup	1 pkg.	0	1	1
broccoli-cheese, w/ham	Hormel Micro Cup	1 pkg.	0	1	4
broccoli-cheese, and rice	Uncle Ben's Hearty	1 pkg.	1	3	1
chicken	Campbell's Instant	1 pkg.	0	2	1
chicken, cream of	Cup-a-Soup	1 pkg.	0	1	1
chicken, hearty, supreme	Cup-a-Soup	1 pkg.	0	1	1
chicken noodle	Cup-a-Soup	1 pkg.	0	1	0
chicken noodle, hearty	Cup-a-Soup	1 pkg.	1	1	1
chicken noodle	Hormel Micro Cup	1 pkg.	1	2	1
chicken, rice	Hormel Micro Cup	1 pkg.	1	3	1
chicken, vegetable	Smart Soup	1 pkg.	2	3	0
chili, hearty	Fantastic Cha-Cha Cup	1 pkg.	1	3	2
clam chowder, New England	Hormel Micro Cup	1 pkg.	1	2	2
corn chowder	Knorr Cup	1 pkg.	0	3	1

PREPARED MEAL ITEM	SPECIFICATIONS	BRAND NAME	SERVING SIZE	PROTEIN BLOCKS	CARBOHYDRATE BLOCKS	FAT BLOCKS
Soup, frozen (cont'd)	corn chowder	Smart Soup	1 pkg.	0	2	0
	corn chowder and potato, creamy	Fantastic Cup	1 pkg.	1	4	0
	corn chowder w/tomatoes	Health Valley	1/2 cup	0	2	0
	couscous	Casbah Moroccan Stew Cup	1 pkg.	1	4	0
	couscous, w/lentil, hearty	Fantastic Cup	1 pkg.	1	4	0
	gumbo, New Orleans	Campbell's Soupsations	1 pkg.	0	4	1
	lentil	Smart Soup	1 pkg.	1	3	0
	lentil, hearty	Campbell's Soup/Recipe	1 pkg.	0	4	1
	lentil, hearty	Campbell's Soupsations	1 pkg.	0	4	5
	lentil, hearty	Fantastic Country Cup	1 pkg.	2	3	0
	lentil, hearty	Knorr Cup	1 pkg.	1	4	0
	lentil, w/couscous	Health Valley	1/3 cup	1	3	0
	minestrone	Smart Soup	1 pkg.	0	2	0
	minestrone, hearty	Fantastic Cup	1 pkg.	1	3	0
	minestrone, hearty	Knorr Cup	1 pkg.	0	3	0

Food	Product	Serving	P	C	F
mushroom, cream of	Cup-a-Soup	1 pkg.	0	1	1
mushroom, creamy	Fantastic Cup	1 pkg.	1	2	0
noodle	Nissin Top Ramen Damae	1 pkg.	0	3	3
noodle	Nissin Top Ramen Oriental	1 pkg.	0	3	3
noodle, chicken free	Fantastic Cup	1 pkg.	1	2	0
noodle, Oriental	Campbell's Ramen Low Fat	1 pkg.	0	5	1
noodle, ring noodle	Cup-a-Soup	1 pkg.	0	1	0
noodle, beef	Campbell's Instant	1 pkg.	0	2	1
noodle, beef	Campbell's Ramen Fried Cup	1 pkg.	2	4	4
noodle, beef	Campbell's Ramen Low Fat	1 pkg.	0	5	1
noodle, beef	Nissin Cup Noodles	1 pkg.	1	4	4
noodle, beef	Nissin Top Ramen	1 pkg.	0	3	3
noodle, beef	Nissin Top Ramen Low Fat	1 pkg.	0	3	0
noodle, beef, onion	Nissin Cup Noodles	1 pkg.	1	4	4
noodle, beef, spicy	Nissin Top Ramen	1 pkg.	0	3	3
noodle, chicken	Campbell's Ramen	1 pkg.	2	4	4
noodle, chicken	Campbell's Ramen Low Fat	1 pkg.	0	5	0
noodle, chicken	Campbell's/Sanwa Ramen	1 pkg.	2	4	4

PREPARED MEAL ITEM	SPECIFICATIONS	BRAND NAME	SERVING SIZE	PROTEIN BLOCKS	CARBOHYDRATE BLOCKS	FAT BLOCKS
Soup, frozen *(cont'd)*	noodle, chicken	Knorr Cup	1 pkg.	0	2	1
	noodle, chicken	Nissin Cup Noodles	1 pkg.	1	4	4
	noodle, chicken	Nissin Top Ramen	1 pkg.	0	3	3
	noodle, chicken	Nissin Top Ramen Low Fat	1 pkg.	0	3	0
	noodle, chicken, broth	Campbell's Instant	1 pkg.	0	2	1
	noodle, chicken, curry	Sanwa Ramen Pride	1 pkg.	2	4	5
	noodle, chicken, mushroom	Nissin Cup Noodles	1 pkg.	1	4	4
	noodle, chicken, mushroom	Nissin Top Ramen	1 pkg.	0	3	3
	noodle, chicken, sesame	Nissin Top Ramen	1 pkg.	0	3	3
	noodle, chicken, spicy	Nissin Cup Noodles	1 pkg.	1	4	4
	noodle, crab	Nissin Cup Noodles	1 pkg.	1	4	4
	noodle, lobster	Nissin Cup Noodles	1 pkg.	1	4	2
	noodle, pork	Campbell's Ramen Low Fat	1 pkg.	0	5	1
	noodle, pork	Nissin Cup Noodles	1 pkg.	1	4	4
	noodle, pork	Nissin Top Ramen	1 pkg.	0	3	3
	noodle, shrimp	Campbell's Ramen	1 pkg.	2	4	5

noodle, shrimp	Campbell's Ramen Low Fat	1 pkg.	0	5	0
noodle, shrimp	Nissin Cup Noodles	1 pkg.	1	4	4
noodle, shrimp	Nissin Top Ramen	1 pkg.	0	3	3
noodle, shrimp	Sanwa Ramen Pride	1 pkg.	2	4	5
noodle, shrimp, picante	Nissin Cup Noodles	1 pkg.	1	4	4
noodle, shrimp, Thai	Sanwa Ramen Pride	1 pkg.	2	4	4
noodle, vegetable, beef	Sanwa Ramen Pride	1 pkg.	2	4	4
noodle, vegetable, curry	Fantastic Cup	1 pkg.	1	3	0
noodle, vegetable, egg, in broth	Campbell's Soupsations	1 pkg.	0	3	1
noodle, vegetable, garden	Nissin Cup Noodles	1 pkg.	1	4	4
noodle, vegetable, hearty	Campbell's Instant	1 pkg.	0	3	1
noodle, vegetable, miso	Fantastic Cup	1 pkg.	1	3	0
noodle, vegetable, tomato	Campbell's/Sanwa Ramen Pride	1 pkg.	2	4	5
noodle, vegetable, tomato	Fantastic Cup	1 pkg.	1	3	0
pasta, Italiano	Health Valley Fat Free	1/2 cup	1	3	0
pasta, marinara, Parmesan, or Mediterranean	Health Valley Pasta Cup Fat Free	1/2 cup	1	2	0

PREPARED MEAL ITEM	SPECIFICATIONS	BRAND NAME	SERVING SIZE	PROTEIN BLOCKS	CARBOHYDRATE BLOCKS	FAT BLOCKS
Soup, frozen *(cont'd)*	pasta and bean	Casbah Pasta Fasul	1 pkg.	1	1	0
	pasta and bean	Bean Cuisine Ultima	1 serving	1	2	0
	pea, green	Cup-a-Soup	1 pkg.	0	2	1
	pea, split	Bean Cuisine Thick as Fog	1 serving	1	2	0
	pea, split	Knorr Cup	1 pkg.	1	3	0
	pea, split	Smart Soup	1 pkg.	1	2	0
	pea, split, hearty	Fantastic Cup	1 pkg.	1	3	0
	potato cheese, w/ham	Hormel Micro Cup	1 pkg.	0	2	4
	potato leek	Knorr Cup	1 pkg.	0	3	0
	potato leek	Smart Soup	1 pkg.	1	2	0
	rice	Casbah Thai Yum	1 pkg.	0	3	0
	rice and beans	Casbah La Fiesta	1 pkg.	1	3	0
	rice and beans, black	Uncle Ben's Hearty	1 pkg.	1	2	1
	rice and beans, Cajun	Casbah Jambalaya	1 pkg.	0	3	0
	rice and beans, Cajun	Fantastic Cup	1 pkg.	1	5	1

rice and beans, Caribbean	Fantastic Cup	1 pkg.	1	4	1
rice and beans, curry, Bombay	Fantastic Cup	1 pkg.	1	4	1
rice and beans, Mexican	Campbell's Soupsations	1 pkg.	0	4	1
rice and beans, Northern Italian	Fantastic Cup	1 pkg.	1	5	1
rice and beans, red	Smart Soup	1 pkg.	1	3	0
rice and beans, Szechuan	Fantastic Cup	1 pkg.	1	4	1
rice and beans, Tex-Mex	Fantastic Cup	1 pkg.	1	5	1
tomato	Cup-a-Soup	1 pkg.	0	2	0
tomato, basil	Uncle Ben's Hearty	1 pkg.	0	2	1
tomato, rice Parmesano	Fantastic Cup	1 pkg.	1	4	1
tomato, vegetable	Campbell's Soupsations	1 pkg.	0	3	1
vegetable, barley, hearty	Fantastic Cup	1 pkg.	1	3	0
vegetable, chicken flavor	Cup-a-Soup	1 pkg.	0	1	0
vegetable, chicken flavor	Knorr Cup	1 pkg.	0	2	0
vegetable, chicken flavor, creamy	Cup-a-Soup	1 pkg.	0	1	1

PREPARED MEAL ITEM	SPECIFICATIONS	BRAND NAME	SERVING SIZE	PROTEIN BLOCKS	CARBOHYDRATE BLOCKS	FAT BLOCKS
Spaghetti dinner	and meatballs, frozen	Swanson	1 pkg.	3	3	4
Spaghetti dishes, mix	w/meat sauce	Kraft Dinner	5 oz.	2	5	4
	mild	Kraft American Dinner	2 oz.	1	4	1
	tangy	Kraft Italian Dinner	2 oz.	1	4	1
Spaghetti entree, canned		Franco-American Garfield Pizzos	1 cup	0	4	1
	w/beef	Franco-American Garfield Pizzos	1 cup	2	3	4
	w/franks	Franco-American SpaghettiO's	1 cup	2	3	4
	w/franks	Van Camp's Weenee	1 can	1	4	3
	w/franks, rings	Kid's Kitchen	7 1/2 oz.	1	4	2
	w/meatballs	Campbell's Superiore/ Franco-American	1 cup	2	3	3
	w/meatballs	Franco-American SpaghettiO's	1 cup	2	3	4
	w/meatballs	Hormel Micro Cup	7 1/2 oz.	1	3	2
	w/meatballs	Libby's Diner	7 3/4 oz.	0	3	2

	w/meatballs	Top Shelf	10 oz.	2	4	4
	w/meatballs, mini meatballs	Kid's Kitchen	7 1/2 oz.	2	3	3
	w/meatballs, rings	Kid's Kitchen	7 1/2 oz.	2	4	2
	rings	Kid's Kitchen	7 1/2 oz.	1	4	1
	tomato-cheese sauce	Franco-American	1 cup	0	4	1
	tomato-cheese sauce	Franco-American SpaghettiO's	1 cup	0	4	1
Spaghetti entree, freeze-dried	w/meat, sauce	Mountain House	1 cup	2	3	2
Spaghetti entree, frozen	Bolognese	Banquet	1 pkg.	2	4	5
	Bolognese	Healthy Choice	1 pkg.	2	4	1
	marinara	Marie Callender's	1 pkg.	1	4	3
	w/meat sauce	The Budget Gourmet Light & Healthy	1 pkg.	2	5	2
	w/meat sauce	Lean Cuisine	1 pkg.	2	5	2
	w/meat sauce	Morton	1 pkg.	1	3	1
	w/meat sauce	Stouffer's Lunch Express	1 pkg.	2	4	3
	w/meat sauce	Weight Watchers	1 pkg.	2	4	2

PREPARED MEAL ITEM	SPECIFICATIONS	BRAND NAME	SERVING SIZE	PROTEIN BLOCKS	CARBOHYDRATE BLOCKS	FAT BLOCKS
Spaghetti entree, frozen *(cont'd)*	w/meatballs	Lean Cuisine	1 pkg.	2	4	2
	w/meatballs	Stouffer's	1 pkg.	3	5	5
Spinach dishes, frozen	au gratin	The Budget Gourmet Side Dish	5 1/2 oz.	1	1	4
	creamed	Green Giant	1/2 cup	1	1	1
	creamed	Seabrook	1/2 cup	1	1	2
	creamed	Stouffer's Side Dish	9-oz. pkg.	2	2	8
	creamed	Tabatchnik	7 1/2 oz.	0	1	1
	feta pocket	Amy's	1 pc.	1	3	2
	Indian	Deep Palak Paneer	5 oz.	1	0	6
	souffle	Stouffer's Side Dish	4 oz.	1	0	3
Stir-fry entree, frozen	lo-mein	Green Giant Create a Meal!	2 1/3 cups, as packaged	1	3	0
	lo-mein	Green Giant Create a Meal!	1 1/4 cups, prepared	5	3	2
	sweet and sour	Green Giant Create a Meal!	2 3/4 cups, as packaged	0	3	0

sweet and sour	Green Giant Create a Meal!	1 1/4 cups, prepared	4	3	2
Szechuan	Green Giant Create a Meal!	2 3/4 cups, as packaged	1	2	2
Szechuan	Green Giant Create a Meal!	1 1/4 cups, prepared	4	2	5
teriyaki	Green Giant Create a Meal!	2 3/4 cups, as packaged	1	2	0
teriyaki	Green Giant Create a Meal!	1 1/4 cups, prepared	4	2	2
teriyaki	Lean Cuisine Lunch Express	9 oz.	2	4	2
vegetable almond	Green Giant Create a Meal!	2 3/4 cups, as packaged	1	2	2
vegetable almond	Green Giant Create a Meal!	1 1/3 cups, prepared	5	2	4
Tamale, canned	Gebhardt	2 pcs.	1	2	7
	Gebhardt Jumbo	2 pcs.	1	2	8

PREPARED MEAL ITEM	SPECIFICATIONS	BRAND NAME	SERVING SIZE	PROTEIN BLOCKS	CARBOHYDRATE BLOCKS	FAT BLOCKS
Tamale, canned		Just Rite	3 pcs.	1	2	6
(cont'd)		Nalley's	3 pcs.	1	3	6
		Old El Paso	3 pcs.	1	3	6
		Van Camp's	2 pcs.	1	2	4
	beef	Hormel	7 1/2-oz. can	1	2	7
	beef, hot-spicy or regular	Hormel	3 pcs.	2	2	7
	beef, jumbo	Hormel	2 pcs.	1	2	7
	chicken	Hormel	3 pcs.	1	2	3
Tamale, frozen		Goya	1 pc.	1	3	6
Tamale pie	Mexican, frozen	Amy's	8 oz.	1	3	1
Tortellini dishes	cheese, frozen	The Budget Gourmet Side Dish	6 oz.	1	2	3
Tortellini entree, canned	cheese	Chef Boyardee	1 cup	1	5	0
	cheese	Franco-American	1 cup	1	5	1
	meat	Chef Boyardee	1 cup	1	5	1
	meat	Franco-American	1 cup	2	4	3

			Protein	Carbohydrate	Fat
Tuna casserole, frozen, noodle	ground beef	Chef Boyardee	7 1/2 oz.	1	4	1
		Stouffer's	1 pkg.	3	4	3
Turkey dinner, frozen	breast	Swanson	1 pkg.	2	4	4
	breast, w/pasta	Weight Watchers	1 pkg.	2	4	2
	breast, stuffed	Healthy Choice	1 pkg.	3	4	1
		Swanson	1 pkg.	2	3	2
		The Budget Gourmet Light & Healthy	1 pkg.	3	2	2
	mostly white meat	Swanson	1 pkg.	1	4	2
	mostly white meat	Swanson Hungry Man	1 pkg.	3	6	5
	and gravy, w/dressing	Banquet	1 pkg.	5	6	7
	and gravy, w/dressing	Marie Callender's	1 pkg.	5	5	6
	gravy and dressing	Dinty Moore American Classics	10 oz.	3	3	3
Turkey entree, canned	gravy and dressing	Libby's Diner	7 oz.	2	2	2
	stew	Dinty Moore	1 cup	1	2	1

PREPARED MEAL ITEM	SPECIFICATIONS	BRAND NAME	SERVING SIZE	PROTEIN BLOCKS	CARBOHYDRATE BLOCKS	FAT BLOCKS
Turkey entree, canned (cont'd)	stew	Dinty Moore Cup	7 1/2 oz.	1	2	1
Turkey entree, freeze-dried	tetrazzini	Mountain House	1 cup	2	2	3
Turkey entree, frozen		Lean Cuisine Homestyle	1 pkg.	3	3	2
	breast, stuffed	Weight Watchers	1 pkg.	2	2	2
	fettuccine alla crema	Healthy Choice	1 pkg.	4	5	1
	glazed	The Budget Gourmet Light & Healthy	1 pkg.	2	4	1
	glazed	Lean Cuisine Café Classics	1 pkg.	2	3	2
	and gravy, w/dressing	Banquet Homestyle	1 pkg.	2	3	3
		Swanson	1 pkg.	1	3	2
	gravy and	Banquet Family	2 slices	1	0	3
	gravy and	Banquet Toppers	5-oz. bag	1	1	1

gravy and w/dressing	Morton	1 pkg.	2	2	3
medallions	Smart Ones	1 pkg.	1	3	1
pie or pot pie	Banquet	1 pkg.	1	4	7
pie or pot pie	Empire Kosher	1 pkg.	3	4	8
pie or pot pie	Lean Cuisine	1 pkg.	3	3	3
pie or pot pie	Marie Callender's	1 pkg.	2	6	15
pie or pot pie	Stouffer's	1 pkg.	3	4	11
pie or pot pie	Swanson	1 pkg.	5	5	8
pie or pot pie	Swanson Hungry Man	1 pkg.	7	7	11
pie or pot pie	Tyson	1 pkg.	2	5	11
open face, w/potato	The Budget Gourmet	1 pkg.	2	3	5
roast	Healthy Choice Country Inn	1 pkg.	4	3	1
roast, breast, and stuffing	Lean Cuisine	1 pkg.	2	5	1
roast, w/mushrooms	Healthy Choice Country	1 pkg.	3	3	1
roast, and stuffing	Stouffer's Homestyle	1 pkg.	3	3	4
tetrazzini	Stouffer's	1 pkg.	3	4	8

PREPARED MEAL ITEM	SPECIFICATIONS	BRAND NAME	SERVING SIZE	PROTEIN BLOCKS	CARBOHYDRATE BLOCKS	FAT BLOCKS
Turkey sandwich, frozen	w/broccoli	Mrs. Paterson's Aussie Pie	1 pc.	2	4	9
	w/broccoli and cheese	Lean Pockets	1 pc.	2	3	3
	and ham w/cheddar	Hot Pockets	1 pc.	2	4	4
	and ham w/cheddar	Lean Pockets	1 pc.	2	3	2
Veal dinner, parmigiana, frozen		Swanson	1 pkg.	4	4	6
Veal entree, parmigiana, frozen		Swanson Hungry Man	1 pkg.	5	7	8
		Banquet	9 oz.	2	3	5
		Morton	9 oz.	1	3	4
		Swanson	1 pkg.	3	3	4
	w/spaghetti	Stouffer's Homestyle	12 oz.	3	4	6
	patties	Banquet Family	1 patty	1	2	5

				P	C	F
Vegetable dinner, frozen	loaf	Amy's Country	1 pkg.	2	6	4
	loaf	Amy's	1 pkg.	1	4	2
	curry	Patak's	1/2 cup	1	2	3
Vegetable entree, frozen	Chinese, and chicken	The Budget Gourmet Light & Healthy	1 pkg.	0	4	3
	country, and beef	Lean Cuisine	1 pkg.	2	3	1
	Italian, and chicken	The Budget Gourmet Light & Healthy	1 pkg.	1	5	2
	pilaf, Indian	Deep	1 cup	1	5	1
	pot pie	Amy's	1 pkg.	1	4	6
	pot pie	Amy's Nondairy	1 pkg.	1	5	3
	pot pie, w/beef	Morton	1 pkg.	1	4	6
	pot pie, w/cheese	Banquet	1 pkg.	1	5	6
	pot pie, w/chicken	Morton	1 pkg.	1	3	6
	pot pie, w/turkey	Morton	1 pkg.	1	3	6
	Shepherd's pie, nondairy	Amy's	1 pkg.	1	2	1
Vegetable entree mix	stew	Knorr	1 pkg.	1	3	1

PREPARED MEAL ITEM	SPECIFICATIONS	BRAND NAME	SERVING SIZE	PROTEIN BLOCKS	CARBOHYDRATE BLOCKS	FAT BLOCKS
Vegetable pocket, frozen, see also specific listings	Bar-B-Q	Ken & Robert's Veggie Pockets	1 pc.	1	4	3
	Greek	Ken & Robert's Veggie Pockets	1 pc.	1	4	3
	Indian	Ken & Robert's Veggie Pockets	1 pc.	1	4	3
	Oriental	Ken & Robert's Veggie Pockets	1 pc.	1	4	3
	pot pie	Amy's	1 pc.	1	4	2
	pot pie	Ken & Robert's Veggie Pockets	1 pc.	1	4	3
	Santa Fe	Ken & Robert's Veggie Pockets	1 pc.	1	4	3
	Tex-Mex	Ken & Robert's Veggie Pockets	1 pc.	1	4	3
Vegetarian entree, see also specific listings	canned	Loma Linda Swiss Stake	1 pc.	1	0	2
	canned, choplet	Worthington	2 pcs.	2	0	1
	canned, cuts, dinner	Loma Linda Swiss Stake	2 pcs.	2	0	1

			Protein	Carbohydrate	Fat
canned, cutlet	Worthington	1 pc.	2	0	0
canned, cutlet, multigrain	Worthington 20 oz.	2 pcs.	2	0	1
canned, cutlet, multigrain	Worthington 50 oz.	1 pc.	2	0	1
frozen	Worthington FriPats	1 patty	2	0	2
frozen	Worthington Stakelets	1 pc.	2	0	3
frozen, croquettes	Worthington Golden	4 pcs.	2	1	3
frozen, dinner entree	Natural Touch	3-oz. patty	3	0	5
frozen, nuggets, w/rice	Hain Hawaiian	10 oz.	2	5	2

PART V

Zone Food Blocks for Fast Foods

More than 50 percent of all meals are now eaten outside the home, and the majority of those come from fast-food restaurants. As you can see in this section, most fast-food meals are both carbohydrate-rich and overloaded with fat—a deadly combination. The excess carbohydrate will rapidly increase insulin levels which then drives the excess fat into storage in your adipose tissue. But by using the Zone Food Blocks, you can go into any fast-food outlet and, by picking and choosing (and discarding most of the excess carbohydrates), make a reasonably good Zone meal.

If you think the packaged food industry has learned that adding more fat makes their grains and starches taste better, then the fast food industry has been an excellent student at learning this valuable lesson. Fat is what makes any meal taste better, and this is why you are going to see that fast foods really load it on to make an otherwise less than appealing food selection seem so wondrous to your taste buds. Just like the food giants, the fast food industry has learned to use grains and starches to keep their costs down. That's why it is such an economic incentive for them to give you super-sized meals. It costs them only pennies more, but you think you're getting a great deal. The only thing you are really getting is more insulin secretion, and that's what makes you fat and keeps you fat.

FOOD ITEM	SPECIFICATIONS	PROTEIN BLOCKS	CARBOHYDRATE BLOCKS	FAT BLOCKS
ARBY'S				
Breakfasts				
bacon	2 strips	1	0	2
biscuit, plain		1	4	5
blueberry muffin		0	4	3
cinnamon–nut danish		1	7	4
croissant, plain		1	3	4
egg portion		0	0	3
French Toastix	6 sticks	1	5	7
ham		1	0	0
sausage		1	0	5
Swiss cheese	1 oz.	2	0	2
table syrup		0	3	0

FAST FOOD RESTAURANT FOOD ITEM	SPECIFICATIONS	PROTEIN BLOCKS	CARBOHYDRATE BLOCKS	FAT BLOCKS
ARBY'S				
Lunch items				
chicken fingers	2 pieces	2	2	5
chicken sandwich	breaded fillet	4	5	9
	Cordon Blue	5	5	11
	grilled, deluxe	3	4	7
	grilled, BBQ	3	5	4
	roast, club	4	4	10
	roast, deluxe, light	3	3	2
	roast, deluxe, sesame seed bun	3	4	7
	roast, Santa Fe	4	4	7
sandwich, ham 'n cheese		3	4	5
sandwich, ham 'n cheese melt		3	4	4
sandwich, fish fillet		3	5	9

sandwich, roast beef	Arby's Melt w/cheddar	3	4	6
sandwich, roast beef	Arby's Q	3	5	6
sandwich, roast beef	Bac'n Cheddar deluxe	3	4	11
sandwich, roast beef	Beef'n Cheddar	4	4	9
sandwich, roast beef	deluxe, light	3	3	3
sandwich, roast beef	giant	5	4	9
sandwich, roast beef	junior	2	4	5
sandwich, roast beef	regular	3	3	6
sandwich, roast beef	super	4	5	9
sandwich, roast turkey deluxe	light	3	3	2
sandwich, sub roll	French dip	4	4	7
sandwich, sub roll	hot Ham'n Swiss	4	5	8
sandwich, sub roll	Italian sub	4	5	12
sandwich, sub roll	Philly Beef'n Swiss	6	5	16
sandwich, sub roll	roast beef sub	5	4	14
sandwich, sub roll	triple cheese melt	5	5	15
sandwich, sub roll	turkey sub	4	5	9
salads	garden	0	1	0

FAST FOOD RESTAURANT

FOOD ITEM	SPECIFICATIONS	PROTEIN BLOCKS	CARBOHYDRATE BLOCKS	FAT BLOCKS
ARBY'S				
salads	roast chicken	3	1	1
salads	side salad	0	0	0
soups	Boston clam chowder	1	2	3
soups	broccoli, cream of	1	1	3
soups	cheese, Wisconsin	1	2	6
soups	chicken noodle	1	1	1
soups	chili, timberline	3	1	3
soups	potato w/bacon	1	2	2
soups	vegetable, lumberjack	0	1	1
potatoes, baked	plain 11 1/2 oz.	1	8	0
potatoes, baked	w/margarine and sour cream	1	9	8
potatoes, baked	Broccoli 'n Cheddar	2	9	7
potatoes, baked	deluxe	3	9	12
potato cakes	2 pcs.	0	2	4

fries	curly	1	4	5
fries	cheddar curly	1	4	6
fries	french	0	3	4
sauces/dressings	Arby's Sauce	0	0	0
sauces/dressings	barbecue sauce	0	1	0
sauces/dressings	beef stock au jus	0	0	0
sauces/dressings	blue cheese dressing	0	0	10
sauces/dressings	buttermilk ranch dressing, reduced calorie	0	1	0
sauces/dressings	cheddar dressing	0	0	1
sauces/dressings	honey French dressing	0	2	8
sauces/dressings	honey mayonnaise, reduced calorie	0	0	2
sauces/dressings	Horsey Sauce	0	0	2
sauces/dressings	Italian dressing, reduced calorie	0	0	0
sauces/dressings	Italian sub sauce	0	0	2
sauces/dressings	mayonnaise	0	0	4
sauces/dressings	mayonnaise, light	0	0	0
sauces/dressings	Parmesan sauce	0	0	2
sauces/dressings	red ranch dressing	0	1	2

FAST FOOD RESTAURANT

FOOD ITEM	SPECIFICATIONS	PROTEIN BLOCKS	CARBOHYDRATE BLOCKS	FAT BLOCKS
ARBY'S				
sauces/dressings	tartar sauce	0	0	5
sauces/dressings	Thousand Island dressing	0	1	9
Desserts and shakes				
apple turnover		1	5	5
cheesecake, plain		1	3	8
cherry turnover		1	5	4
chocolate chip cookie		0	2	2
Polar Swirl	Butterfinger	2	7	6
Polar Swirl	Heath	2	8	7
Polar Swirl	Oreo	2	7	7
Polar Swirl	Snickers	2	8	6
Polar Swirl	peanut butter cup	3	7	8
shake	chocolate	2	8	4

shake	jamocha	2	7	3
shake	vanilla	2	6	4

BURGER KING

Breakfasts

biscuit	w/bacon, egg, cheese	3	4	10
biscuit	w/sausage	2	4	13
Croissan'wich	sausage, egg, cheese	3	3	15
French toast sticks		1	7	9
hash browns		0	3	4

Lunch items

BK Big Fish		4	6	14
BK Broiler chicken		4	4	10
cheeseburger	regular	3	3	6
cheeseburger	double	6	3	12
cheeseburger	double w/bacon	6	3	13
chicken sandwich		4	6	14

FAST FOOD RESTAURANT FOOD ITEM	SPECIFICATIONS	PROTEIN BLOCKS	CARBOHYDRATE BLOCKS	FAT BLOCKS
BURGER KING				
Double Whopper	regular	7	5	19
Double Whopper	w/cheese	7	5	21
hamburger		3	3	18
Whopper		4	5	13
Whopper	w/cheese	5	5	15
Whopper Jr.		3	3	8
Whopper Jr.	w/cheese	3	3	9
Chicken Tenders	6 pcs.	2	1	4
dipping sauces 1 oz.	A.M. Express	0	2	0
dipping sauces 1 oz.	barbecue sauce	0	1	0
dipping sauces 1 oz.	Bull's Eye	0	1	0
dipping sauces 1 oz.	honey	0	3	0
dipping sauces 1 oz.	ranch	0	0	6
dipping sauces 1 oz.	sweet and sour	0	1	0

Side dishes

fries, medium		1	4	7
onion rings		1	4	5
salad, w/out dressing	chicken, broiled	3	0	3
salad, w/out dressing	garden	0	0	2
salad, w/out dressing	side	0	0	1

Salad dressings ½ oz.

blue cheese	0	0	5
French	0	1	3
Italian, light	0	0	0
ranch	0	0	6
Thousand Island	0	1	4

Desserts and shakes

Dutch apple pie	0	4	5
shakes, medium	chocolate	1	6	2
shakes, medium	chocolate, w/syrup	1	9	2

FAST FOOD RESTAURANT FOOD ITEM	SPECIFICATIONS	PROTEIN BLOCKS	CARBOHYDRATE BLOCKS	FAT BLOCKS
BURGER KING				
shakes, medium	strawberry, w/syrup	1	9	2
shakes, medium	vanilla	1	6	2
CARL'S JR				
Breakfast 1 serving				
bacon	2 strips	0	0	1
breakfast burrito		3	3	9
English muffin w/margarine		1	3	3
French toast dips	w/out syrup	1	4	8
quesadilla, breakfast		2	3	5
sausage	1 patty	1	0	6
scrambled eggs		2	0	4
Sunrise Sandwich		2	3	7
table syrup	1 oz.	0	2	0

chicken stars			
sauces			
6 pcs.	2	1	5
barbeque	0	1	0
honey sauce	0	3	0
mustard sauce	0	1	0
salsa	0	0	0
sweet'n sour sauce	0	1	0
Lunch Items			
Sandwiches			
Big Burger	4	5	7
Carl's Catch Fish Sandwich	2	5	10
chicken bacon Swiss	4	6	12
chicken, barbeque	4	3	2
chicken club	5	4	10
chicken, ranch	3	6	10
chicken, Santa Fe	4	4	10
double cheeseburger, 1/2 lb.			
double cheeseburger, 1/3 lb.	5	4	14
Double Western Bacon Cheeseburger	8	3	19

FAST FOOD RESTAURANT

FOOD ITEM	SPECIFICATIONS	PROTEIN BLOCKS	CARBOHYDRATE BLOCKS	FAT BLOCKS
CARL'S JR				
	Famous Big Star hamburger	4	4	13
	hamburger	2	2	3
	Hot & Crispy sandwich	2	4	7
	Super Star hamburger	6	4	18
	Western Bacon Cheeseburger	5	6	12
"Great Stuff" potato	bacon and cheese	3	8	10
	broccoli and cheese	2	8	7
	potato, plain	1	7	0
	sour cream and chive	1	7	5
Entree Salads-to-Go	chicken	4	1	3
	garden	0	0	1
salad dressings 2 oz.	blue cheese	0	0	11
	French, fat free	0	2	0
	house	0	0	7

		P	C	F
side dishes	Italian, fat free	0	0	0
	Thousand Island	0	1	8
	CrossCut Fries, large	1	6	11
	fries, regular	1	5	7
	hash brown nuggets	0	3	6
	onion rings	1	7	9
	zucchini	1	4	8
bakery products	blueberry muffin	1	5	5
	bran muffin	1	6	4
	cheese danish	1	5	7
	cheesecake, strawberry swirl	1	3	6
	chocolate cake	0	5	3
	chocolate chip cookie	0	5	6
	cinnamon roll	1	7	4
shake, small	chocolate	1	8	2
	strawberry	1	9	2
	vanilla	2	6	3

FAST FOOD RESTAURANT

FOOD ITEM	SPECIFICATIONS	PROTEIN BLOCKS	CARBOHYDRATE BLOCKS	FAT BLOCKS
CHICK-FIL-A				
chicken dishes	3 1/2 oz.	3	0	3
	chargrilled, 3 oz.	4	0	1
	Chick-fil-A Nuggets, 8 pack	4	1	5
	Chick-n-Strips, 4 pcs.	4	1	3
	Chick-n-Strips Salad	5	2	3
	salad, chargrilled garden	4	1	1
	salad plate	3	4	2
chicken sandwiches	regular	3	3	3
	chargrilled	4	4	1
	chargrilled, deluxe	4	4	1
	chargrilled club, w/out dressing	5	4	4
	Chick-n-Q	4	4	4
	deluxe	4	3	3
	salad, whole wheat	4	5	2

	P	C	F
side dishes, small			
carrot raisin salad	1	3	1
chicken soup 1 cup	2	1	0
coleslaw	1	1	2
tossed salad	1	1	0
Waffle fries, salted	0	5	3
Waffle fries, unsalted	0	5	3
desserts			
brownies, fudge nut	1	5	5
cheesecake	2	1	7
cheesecake, w/blueberry	2	1	8
cheesecake, w/strawberry	2	1	8
Icedream, small cone	2	2	1
Icedream, small cup	2	6	3
lemon pie	0	2	7

CHURCH'S CHICKEN

	P	C	F
chicken, edible portion			
breast 2.8 oz.	3	0	4
leg 2 oz.	2	0	3

FOOD ITEM	SPECIFICATIONS	PROTEIN BLOCKS	CARBOHYDRATE BLOCKS	FAT BLOCKS
CHURCH'S CHICKEN				
	Tender Strip 1.1 oz.	1	0	1
	thigh 3 oz.	2	1	5
	wing 3 oz.	3	1	5
	biscuit	0	3	5
	Cajun rice	0	2	2
	coleslaw	1	1	2
	corn on cob	1	2	1
sides	fries	0	3	4
	okra	0	2	5
	potatoes and gravy	0	1	1
apple pie		0	4	4

DAIRY QUEEN/BRAZIER

DQ Homestyle burgers

cheeseburger	3	3	6
double cheeseburger	5	3	10
deluxe double cheeseburger	5	3	10
cheeseburger w/bacon, double	6	3	12
hamburger	2	3	4
hamburger, deluxe, double	4	3	7
Ultimate burger	6	3	14

Sandwiches

chicken fillet, breaded	3	4	7
breaded w/cheese	4	4	8
grilled	3	3	3
fish fillet	2	4	5
fish fillet w/cheese	3	4	7
hot dog, plain	1	2	5

FAST FOOD RESTAURANT				
FOOD ITEM	SPECIFICATIONS	PROTEIN BLOCKS	CARBOHYDRATE BLOCKS	FAT BLOCKS
DAIRY QUEEN/BRAZIER				
	w/cheese	2	2	6
	w/chili	2	2	5
	w/chili and cheese	2	2	7
chicken strip basket	w/gravy	5	9	14
	w/BBQ sauce	5	9	12
Side dishes				
fries	large	1	5	6
	regular	1	4	5
	small	0	3	3
onion rings	regular	1	3	4
Desserts and shakes				
banana split		1	10	4
Blizzard	Butterfinger, regular	2	13	9

Butterfinger, small	2	9	6
chocolate chip cookie dough, regular	2	16	12
chocolate chip cookie dough, small	2	11	8
chocolate sandwich cookie, regular	2	11	8
chocolate sandwich cookie, small	1	9	6
Heath, regular	2	13	11
Heath, small	1	9	7
Reese's peanut butter cup, regular	3	11	11
Reese's peanut butter cup, small	2	9	8
strawberry, regular	2	10	5
strawberry, small	1	7	4
Buster Bar	1	4	9
cone, chocolate			
regular	1	6	4
small	1	4	3
cone, chocolate-dipped			
regular	1	7	8
small	1	5	6
cone, vanilla			
large	1	7	4
regular	1	6	3

FAST FOOD RESTAURANT

FOOD ITEM	SPECIFICATIONS	PROTEIN BLOCKS	CARBOHYDRATE BLOCKS	FAT BLOCKS
DAIRY QUEEN/BRAZIER				
	small	1	4	2
DQ cake, undecorated	heart	10	40	30
	log	10	40	24
	round, 8"	8	48	32
	round, 10"	12	72	48
	sheet	20	120	80
DQ caramel & nut bar		1	4	4
DQ fudge bar		1	1	0
DQ Lemon Freez'r	1/2 cup	0	2	0
DQ sandwich		0	3	2
DQ Treatzza Pizza 1/8 pie	Heath	0	3	2
	M & M	0	3	2
	peanut butter fudge	1	3	3
	strawberry–banana	0	3	2

		P	C	F
DQ vanilla orange bar		0	2	0
Dilly bar	chocolate	0	2	4
	chocolate mint	0	2	4
	toffee, w/Heath	0	3	4
Fudge Nut bar	regular	1	4	8
malt, chocolate	regular	3	17	7
	small	2	12	5
Misty	cooler, strawberry	0	5	0
	slush, regular	0	8	0
	slush, small	0	6	0
Peanut Buster parfait		2	11	10
Queen's Choice Big Scoop	chocolate	1	3	5
	vanilla	1	3	5
shake, chocolate	regular	2	14	7
	small	2	10	5
soft-serve, DQ	chocolate, 1/2 cup	1	2	2
	vanilla, 1/2 cup	0	2	2
Starkiss		0	2	0

FAST FOOD RESTAURANT

FOOD ITEM	SPECIFICATIONS	PROTEIN BLOCKS	CARBOHYDRATE BLOCKS	FAT BLOCKS
DAIRY QUEEN/BRAZIER				
strawberry shortcake		1	8	5
sundae, chocolate	regular	1	8	3
	small	1	6	2
yogurt, Breeze	Heath, regular	2	14	6
	Heath, small	2	9	3
	strawberry, regular	2	11	3
	strawberry, small	1	7	0
	DQ Nonfat 1/2 cup	0	2	0
yogurt, frozen	regular cup	1	5	0
	cone	1	7	0
	strawberry sundae	1	7	0

DOMINO'S PIZZA

1/4 of 12" pie (2 slices) except as noted

deep dish			
	cheese	3	7	8
	ham	4	7	8
	pepperoni	4	7	10
	sausage and mushroom	4	7	9
	veggie	3	7	12
	X-tra cheese and pepperoni	4	7	11
hand tossed	cheese	2	5	3
	ham	2	5	3
	pepperoni	3	5	5
	sausage and mushroom	3	5	5
	veggie	2	5	3
	X-tra cheese and pepperoni	3	5	6
thin crust, 1/3 pie	cheese	2	4	5
	ham	3	4	6
	pepperoni	3	4	8

FAST FOOD RESTAURANT

FOOD ITEM	SPECIFICATIONS	PROTEIN BLOCKS	CARBOHYDRATE BLOCKS	FAT BLOCKS
DOMINO'S PIZZA				
	sausage and mushroom	3	5	7
	veggie	2	4	6
	X-tra cheese and pepperoni	3	4	9
JACK-IN-THE-BOX				
Breakfast				
Breakfast Jack		3	3	4
croissant	sausage	3	4	16
	supreme	3	4	12
hash browns		0	1	4
jelly, grape	1/2 oz.	0	1	0
pancake platter		2	6	4
pancake syrup	1 1/2 oz.	0	3	0
sandwich, breakfast	sourdough	3	3	7

Sandwiches

scrambled egg pocket	5	4	12
ultimate	4	3	7
Sandwiches			
beef, Monterey roast			
cheeseburger			
regular	4	4	10
double	2	4	5
ultimate	3	4	8
bacon bacon	7	3	26
Colossus	5	5	15
The Outlaw Burger	8	3	28
chicken	4	6	13
chicken, Caesar	3	4	6
chicken, spicy crispy	4	4	9
chicken, supreme	3	6	9
chicken fajita pita	4	5	12
chicken fillet, grilled	3	3	3
The Really Big Chicken Sandwich	6	6	19

FAST FOOD RESTAURANT

FOOD ITEM	SPECIFICATIONS	PROTEIN BLOCKS	CARBOHYDRATE BLOCKS	FAT BLOCKS
JACK-IN-THE-BOX				
fish supreme		3	5	11
hamburger	regular	2	3	4
	quarter-pounder	4	4	9
	sourdough, grilled	5	4	14
Jumbo Jack		4	5	11
Jumbo Jack w/cheese		4	5	13
Entrees				
chicken teriyaki bowl		4	12	1
taco		1	1	4
taco, super		2	2	6
Salads				
chicken, garden		3	1	3
side		1	0	1

Finger foods

chicken strips	4 pcs.	4	2	4
chicken strips	6 pcs.	6	3	7
egg rolls	3 pcs.	0	6	8
egg rolls	5 pcs.	1	9	14
jalapenos, stuffed	7 pcs.	2	3	9
jalapenos, stuffed	10 pcs.	3	4	13
potato wedges w/bacon, cheddar		3	5	19

Side dishes

fries	small	0	3	4
	regular	1	5	6
	jumbo	1	5	6
	super scoop	1	8	10
	seasoned, curly	1	4	7
onion rings		1	4	8

FAST FOOD RESTAURANT

FOOD ITEM	SPECIFICATIONS	PROTEIN BLOCKS	CARBOHYDRATE BLOCKS	FAT BLOCKS
JACK-IN-THE-BOX				
Sauces				
barbeque	1 oz.	0	1	0
buttermilk	1 oz.	0	0	4
soy	1/3 oz.	0	0	0
sweet and sour	1 oz.	0	1	0
tartar	1 oz.	0	0	5
dressings, 2 oz.	blue cheese	0	1	6
	buttermilk, house	0	1	10
	Italian, low calorie	0	0	1
	Thousand Island	0	1	8
Condiments				
cheese 1 slice	American	0	0	1
	Swiss style	0	0	1

croutons	1/2 oz.	0	1	1
guacamole	3/4 oz.	0	0	1
hot sauce pkt.		0	0	0
ketchup pkt.		0	0	0
mayonnaise pkt.		0	0	6
mustard pkt.		0	0	0
mustard pkt., Chinese hot		0	0	0
salsa	1 oz.	0	0	0
sour cream	1 oz.	0	0	2

Desserts

apple turnover		0	5	6
cheesecake		1	3	6
cheesecake, chocolate chip cookie dough		1	5	6
shakes	chocolate	1	8	2
	strawberry	1	7	2
	vanilla	1	7	2

FAST FOOD RESTAURANT FOOD ITEM	SPECIFICATIONS	PROTEIN BLOCKS	CARBOHYDRATE BLOCKS	FAT BLOCKS
KFC				
Original Recipe	breast	5	1	7
	drumstick	2	0	2
	thigh	3	1	6
	wing, whole	2	1	3
Colonel's Rotisserie Gold	breast/wing	6	0	6
	breast/wing, w/out skin	5	0	2
	thigh/leg	4	0	8
	thigh/leg w/out skin	4	0	4
Extra Tasty Crispy	breast	4	3	9
	drumstick	2	1	4
	thigh	3	2	8
	wing/whole	1	1	4
Hot and Spicy	breast	5	2	12
	drumstick	2	1	4

thigh	3	1	9
wing, whole	1	1	5
chicken pot pie	4	7	13
Crispy Strips	4 pcs.	4	1	7
Hot Wings	6 pcs.	4	2	11
Kentucky Nuggets	6 pcs.	2	2	6

Sandwiches

chicken	4	5	7
Colonel's chicken	3	4	9
BBQ chicken	2	3	3

Sides/specials

BBQ baked beans	1	2	1
beans, red, and rice	1	2	1
biscuit	0	2	4
coleslaw	0	1	2
corn-on-the-cob	1	2	4

FAST FOOD RESTAURANT

FOOD ITEM	SPECIFICATIONS	PROTEIN BLOCKS	CARBOHYDRATE BLOCKS	FAT BLOCKS
KFC				
corn bread		0	3	4
garden rice		0	2	0
macaroni & cheese		1	2	3
mashed potato w/gravy		0	2	2
Mean Greens		0	1	1
potato salad		0	2	4
potato wedges		0	2	3
LITTLE CAESARS				
Baby Pan!Pan!	2 sqs.	5	7	8
Crazy Bread		0	2	1
Crazy Sauce	6 oz.	1	1	0
Pan!Pan!, 1 medium slice	cheese only	1	2	2
	pepperoni	2	2	3

		P	C	F
Pizza/Pizza, 1 medium slice	cheese only	2	3	2
	pepperoni	2	3	3
salads, individual	antipasto	2	1	4
	Caesar	1	1	2
	Greek	1	1	3
	tossed	1	2	1
dressings, 1.5 oz.	blue cheese	0	1	5
	Caesar	0	0	9
	French	0	1	5
	Greek	0	0	10
	Italian	0	0	7
	Italian, fat free	0	0	0
	ranch	0	1	7
	Thousand Island	0	1	6
sandwich, cold	ham and cheese	4	8	12
	Italian	4	8	12
	veggie	3	8	10
sandwich, hot	Cheeser	6	8	13

FAST FOOD RESTAURANT FOOD ITEM	SPECIFICATIONS	PROTEIN BLOCKS	CARBOHYDRATE BLOCKS	FAT BLOCKS
LITTLE CAESARS				
	Meatsa	8	8	19
	pepperoni	6	8	16
	supreme	6	8	15
	veggie	5	8	8
LONG JOHN SILVER'S				
clams	3 oz.	2	3	6
chicken	batter-dipped, 1 pc.	1	1	2
	Flavorbaked, 1 pc.	3	0	1
	popcorn, 3 1/3 oz.	2	2	5
fish	batter-dipped, 1 pc.	2	1	4
	Flavorbaked, 1 pc.	2	0	1
	popcorn, 3 1/3 oz.	2	3	5
shrimp	batter-dipped, 1 pc.	0	0	1

	popcorn, 3 1/3 oz.	2	3	5
Sandwiches 1 pc.				
chicken, Flavorbaked		3	3	3
fish, batter-dipped, w/out sauce		2	4	4
fish, Flavorbaked		3	3	5
Ultimate Fish		3	5	7
Sides, 1 serving				
cheese sticks	1 1/2 oz.	1	1	3
coleslaw		0	2	2
corn cobbette, 1 pc.	w/butter	0	2	3
	plain	0	2	0
fries	3 oz.	0	3	5
green beans		0	0	0
hushpuppy	1 pc.	0	1	1
potato	baked	1	5	0
rice pilaf		0	3	2
side salad		0	0	0

FAST FOOD RESTAURANT FOOD ITEM	SPECIFICATIONS	PROTEIN BLOCKS	CARBOHYDRATE BLOCKS	FAT BLOCKS
LONG JOHN SILVER'S				
Dressings				
French	fat free, 1 1/2 oz.	0	2	0
Italian	1 oz.	0	0	5
ranch	1 oz.	0	0	6
	fat free, 1 1/2 oz.	0	1	0
Thousand Island	1 oz.	0	1	3
Sauces, condiments				
honey mustard	1/2 oz.	0	1	0
malt vinegar	1/3 oz.	0	0	0
margarine	1/5 oz.	0	0	1
shrimp sauce	1/2 oz.	0	0	0
sour cream	1 oz.	0	0	2
sweet 'n' sour	1/2 oz.	0	1	0

	tartar sauce (1/2 oz.)	0	1	1

MCDONALD'S

breakfast biscuit	plain	1	3	4
	bacon, egg, and cheese	2	4	8
	sausage	1	3	10
	sausage and egg	2	4	12
breakfast burrito		2	2	7
breakfast dishes	eggs, scrambled, 2	2	0	4
	hash browns	0	1	3
	hotcakes, plain	1	6	2
	hotcakes, w/syrup, margarine	1	11	5
	sausage	1	0	5
breakfast muffin	English	1	3	1
	Egg McMuffin	2	3	4
	Sausage McMuffin	2	3	8
	Sausage McMuffin w/egg	3	3	10
danish and muffin	apple bran muffin	1	4	0

FAST FOOD RESTAURANT FOOD ITEM	SPECIFICATIONS	PROTEIN BLOCKS	CARBOHYDRATE BLOCKS	FAT BLOCKS
MCDONALD'S				
	apple danish	1	6	5
	cheese danish	1	5	7
	cinnamon raisin danish	1	6	7
	cinnamon roll	1	5	7
	raspberry danish	1	6	5
Sandwiches				
Arch Deluxe		4	4	10
Arch Deluxe, w/bacon		5	4	11
Big Mac		4	5	9
cheeseburger		2	4	5
Filet-O-Fish		2	4	5
hamburger		2	4	3
McChicken		2	5	10

		Protein	Carbohydrate	Fat
McGrilled Chicken Classic		3	3	1
Quarter Pounder		3	4	7
Quarter Pounder, w/cheese		4	4	7
Chicken McNuggets	4 pcs.	2	1	4
	6 pcs.	3	2	6
	9 pcs.	4	3	9
McNuggets sauce pkt.	barbeque	0	1	0
	honey	0	1	0
	honey mustard	0	0	2
	hot mustard	0	1	1
	sweet and sour	0	1	0
french fries	small	0	3	3
	large	1	6	7
	Super Size	1	7	9
salads	chicken, fajita	3	1	2
	garden	1	1	1
salad bacon bits	1 pkg.	0	0	0
salad croutons	1 pkg.	0	1	1

FAST FOOD RESTAURANT

FOOD ITEM	SPECIFICATIONS	PROTEIN BLOCKS	CARBOHYDRATE BLOCKS	FAT BLOCKS
MCDONALD'S				
salad dressing, 1 pkg.	blue cheese	0	1	6
	ranch	0	1	7
	red French, reduced calorie	0	3	3
	Thousand Island	0	2	4
	vinaigrette, lite	0	1	1
Desserts and shakes				
baked apple pie		0	4	4
McDonaldland Cookies	1 pkg.	1	4	3
shake, small	chocolate	2	7	2
	strawberry	2	7	2
	vanilla	2	7	2
sundae	hot fudge	1	6	2
sundae nuts	1/4 oz.	0	0	1
yogurt, frozen, lowfat	cone, vanilla	1	3	0

hot caramel sundae	1	7	1
strawberry sundae	1	6	0

PIZZA HUT

1 slice of medium pie, except as noted

Bigfoot 1 slice			
cheese	1	3	2
pepperoni	1	3	2
pepperoni, mushroom, and sausage	2	3	3
breadsticks			
5 pcs.	3	14	5
hand-tossed			
cheese	2	3	2
beef	2	3	3
ham	2	3	2
Meat Lovers	2	3	4
pepperoni	2	3	3
Pepperoni Lovers	2	3	0
pork topping	2	3	3
sausage, Italian	2	3	4
supreme	2	3	4

FAST FOOD RESTAURANT

FOOD ITEM	SPECIFICATIONS	PROTEIN BLOCKS	CARBOHYDRATE BLOCKS	FAT BLOCKS
PIZZA HUT				
	supreme, super	2	3	4
	Veggie Lovers	2	3	2
pan pizza	cheese	2	3	4
	beef	2	3	4
	ham	2	3	7
	Meat Lovers	2	3	6
	pepperoni	2	3	4
	Pepperoni Lovers	2	3	6
	pork topping	2	3	5
	sausage, Italian	2	3	5
	supreme	2	3	5
	supreme, super	2	3	6
	Veggie Lovers	1	3	3
Personal Pan Pizza, 1 pie	pepperoni	4	7	9

Thin 'N Crispy

supreme	5	7	11
cheese	2	2	3
beef	2	2	4
ham	1	2	2
Meat Lovers	2	2	4
pepperoni	2	2	3
Pepperoni Lovers	2	2	5
pork topping	2	2	4
sausage, Italian	2	2	4
supreme	2	2	4
supreme, super	2	2	5
Veggie Lovers	1	2	2

SIZZLER

Hot entrees

hamburger on bun w/lettuce, tomato	6	4	11
chicken breast 5 oz.	4	1	1

Zone Food Blocks for Fast Foods • 287

FAST FOOD RESTAURANT

FOOD ITEM	SPECIFICATIONS	PROTEIN BLOCKS	CARBOHYDRATE BLOCKS	FAT BLOCKS
SIZZLER				
hibachi, w/pineapple		4	0	1
Santa Fe		4	0	1
Malibu chicken patty		3	1	6
salmon	8 oz.	5	0	4
shrimp, broiled	5 oz.	3	0	2
shrimp, fried	4 pcs.	3	4	1
shrimp, mini	4 oz.	2	3	0
shrimp scampi	5 oz.	4	0	1
steak, Dakota, ranch	6 oz.	4	0	7
	8 oz.	5	0	9
	9 oz.	7	0	11
swordfish	8 oz.	6	0	5

Side dishes

	Serving			
cheese toast		1	2	7
french fries	4 oz.	1	5	4
potato, baked, pulp		0	2	0
rice pilaf	6 oz.	1	5	2
sauces 1 1/2 oz.	buttery dipping	0	0	12
	cocktail sauce	0	1	0
	hibachi sauce	0	1	0
	Malibu sauce	0	0	10
	sour dressing	0	0	3
	tartar sauce	0	1	6

Hot bar

	Serving			
chicken wings	1 oz.	1	0	7
focaccia bread	2 pcs.	0	1	2
marinara sauce	1 oz.	0	0	0
meatballs	4	1	0	4
nacho sauce	2 oz.	1	0	3

FAST FOOD RESTAURANT

FOOD ITEM	SPECIFICATIONS	PROTEIN BLOCKS	CARBOHYDRATE BLOCKS	FAT BLOCKS
SIZZLER				
pasta, fettuccine	2 oz.	0	2	0
pasta, spaghetti	2 oz.	0	2	0
potato skins	2 oz.	0	2	3
refried beans	1/4 cup	1	1	0
saltines	2 pcs.	0	0	0
taco filling	2 oz.	0	0	3
taco shells	1 pc.	0	1	1
soup, 4 oz.	broccoli, cheese	0	1	3
	chicken noodle soup	0	0	0
	clam chowder	0	1	2
	minestrone soup	0	1	0
	vegetable sirloin	1	1	1

Salads, prepared, 2 oz.

carrot and raisin	0	1	3
Chinese chicken	1	1	1
jicama, spicy	0	0	0
Mediterranean Minted Fruit	0	1	0
Mexican Fiesta	0	1	0
pasta, seafood, Louis	0	1	1
potato, old-fashioned	0	1	2
potato, red herb	0	1	3
seafood Louis	0	0	1
teriyaki beef	1	1	1
tuna pasta	1	1	3

Dressings, 1 oz.

blue cheese	0	0	4
guacamole	0	0	1
honey mustard	0	0	5
Italian, lite	0	0	0

FAST FOOD RESTAURANT FOOD ITEM	SPECIFICATIONS	PROTEIN BLOCKS	CARBOHYDRATE BLOCKS	FAT BLOCKS
SIZZLER				
Parmesan, Italian		0	0	3
ranch		0	0	4
ranch, lite		0	0	3
rice vinegar, Japanese		0	0	0
salsa		0	0	0
sour dressing		0	0	2
Thousand Island		0	0	5
WENDY'S				
Sandwiches				
bacon cheeseburger, Jr.		3	4	7
Big Bacon Classic		5	5	11
cheeseburger	Jr.	2	4	4
	Jr., Deluxe	3	4	5

chicken	Kid's Meal		2	3	4
	grilled		3	4	2
	breaded		4	5	6
	spicy		3	4	7
	club		5	5	8
hamburger	single, plain		4	3	5
	single, everything		4	4	7
	Jr.		2	4	3
	Kid's Meal		2	3	3
Sandwich components					
American cheese	1 slice		0	0	2
American cheese Jr.			0	0	1
bacon			0	0	1
ketchup	1 tsp.		0	0	0
mayonnaise	1 1/2 tsp.		0	0	1
mustard	1/2 tsp.		0	0	0
onion	4 rings		0	0	0

FAST FOOD RESTAURANT

FOOD ITEM	SPECIFICATIONS	PROTEIN BLOCKS	CARBOHYDRATE BLOCKS	FAT BLOCKS
WENDY'S				
pickles	4 slices	0	0	0
chicken nuggets	5 pcs.	2	1	5
nuggets sauce, 1 oz.	barbeque	0	1	0
	honey	0	1	0
	honey mustard	0	1	4
	spicy buffalo wing	0	0	1
	sweet and sour	0	1	0
chili	small, 8 oz.	2	2	2
	large, 12 oz.	3	3	3
	cheddar cheese, shredded, 2 Tbsp.	1	0	2
	saltine crackers, 2	0	0	0
baked potato	plain	1	7	0
	bacon and cheese	2	8	6
	broccoli and cheese	1	8	5

fries	cheese	2	8	8
	chili and cheese	3	8	8
	sour cream w/chive	1	7	2
	small	0	3	4
	medium	1	5	6
	Biggie	1	6	8
Salads-to-go, fresh, w/out dressing	deluxe garden	1	1	2
	grilled chicken	4	1	3
	side salad	1	0	1
	side salad, Caesar	1	1	2
	taco salad	4	5	10
	soft breadstick	1	3	1
dressing, 2 Tbsp.	blue cheese	0	0	6
	French	0	1	3
	French, fat free	0	1	0
	French, sweet red	0	1	3
	Italian, reduced fat/calorie	0	0	1
	Italian, Caesar	0	0	5

FAST FOOD RESTAURANT

FOOD ITEM	SPECIFICATIONS	PROTEIN BLOCKS	CARBOHYDRATE BLOCKS	FAT BLOCKS
WENDY'S				
	ranch, Hidden Valley	0	0	3
	ranch, Hidden Valley, reduced fat/calorie	0	0	2
	Thousand Island	0	0	4
desserts	chocolate chip cookie	1	4	4
	Frosty, small	1	6	3
	Frosty, medium	2	8	4
	Frosty, large	2	10	6

APPENDIX

A. CONTINUING SUPPORT

If you are interested in learning more about the Zone Diet and the food products that make it easier to stay in the Zone, please go to *www.zonediet.com*.

B. ZONE BLOCK HELP

The average female will need meals consisting of three blocks, and the average male will require meals containing four blocks. If you want even more precision, call my toll-free information line (1-800-404-8171), which will provide you with a free analysis of your percent body fat, your lean body mass, and the number of Zone Food Blocks you need per day. Alternatively you can go to my website (*www.drsears.com*) and do it yourself. The analysis only takes a few seconds over the phone, and all the information you need will be sent to you free of charge in a hard copy format.

Make sure you have the following information ready:

Females:

1. Your barefoot height in inches.

2. Your waist measurement in inches at your belly button.

3. Your hip measurement in inches at the widest point.

Males:

1. Your weight in pounds.

2. Your waist measurement in inches at your belly button.

3. Your wrist measurement in inches of your dominant hand just inside your wrist bone.

C. REFERENCES

1. Heini AF and Weinsier RL. "Divergent trends in obesity and fat intake patterns: the American paradox." *Am J Med* 102: 259–264 (1997).

2. Katan MB, Grundy SM, and Willett WC. "Beyond low-fat diets." *N Engl J Med* 337: 563–566 (1997).

3. Jeppesen J, Schaaf P, Jones C, Zhou MY, and Reaven GM. "Effects of low-fat, high-

carbohydrate diets on risk factors for ischemic heart disease in postmenopausal women." *Am J Clin Nutr* 65: 1027–1033 (1997).

4. Liu S and Willett WC. "Dietary glycemic load and atherothrombotic risk." *Current Atheroscler Rep* 4: 454–461 (2002).

5. Liu S, Manson JE, Burning JE, Stampfer, Willett WC, and Ridker PM. "Relation between a diet with a glycemic load and plasma concentrations of high-sensitivity C-reactive protein in middle aged women." *American Journal of Clinical Nutrition*, 75: 492–498 (2002).

6. Albert CM, Hennekens CH, O'Donnell CJ, Ajani UA, Carey VJ, Willett WC, Ruskin JN, and Manson JE. "Fish consumption and risk of sudden death." *JAMA* 279: 23–28 (1998).

7. GISSI investigators. "Dietary supplementation with m-3 polyunsaturated fatty acids and Vitamin E after myocardial infarction." *Lancet* 354: 447–455 (1991).

Additional Books in the Zone

Sears, B., *The Zone*, ReganBooks, NY (1995).

Sears, B., *Mastering the Zone*, ReganBooks, NY (1997).

Sears, B., *Zone Perfect Meals in Minutes*, ReganBooks, NY (1998).

Sears, B., *The Soy Zone*, ReganBooks, NY (2000).

Sears, B., *A Week in the Zone*, ReganBooks, NY (2001).

Sears, B., *The Top 100 Zone Foods*, ReganBooks, NY (2002).

Sears, B., *The Omega Rx Zone*, ReganBooks, NY (2003).

Sears, B., *Zone Meals in Seconds*, ReganBooks, NY (2004).

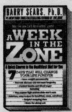
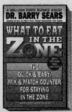

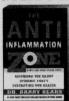